THE END OF DIETING

THE END OF DIETING

How to Live for Life

Joel Fuhrman, M.D.

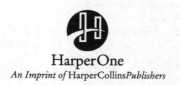

HarperOne
An Imprint of HarperCollins*Publishers*

HarperOne

This book contains advice and information relating to health care. It should be used to supplement rather than replace the advice of your doctor or another trained health professional. If you know or suspect that you have a health problem, it is recommended that you seek your physician's advice before embarking on any medical program or treatment. All efforts have been made to assure the accuracy of the information contained in this book as of the date of publication. The publisher and the author disclaim liability for any medical outcomes that may occur as a result of applying the methods suggested in this book.

FIRST HARPERCOLLINS PAPERBACK EDITION PUBLISHED IN 2015

Interior Design by Laura Lind Design

ISBN 978-0-06-224933-3

Library of Congress Cataloging-in-Publication Data
Fuhrman, Joel.
 The End of Dieting : How to Live for Life / Joel Fuhrman, M.D.—First edition.
  pages cm
Includes bibliographical references and index.
ISBN 978–0–06–224932–6 (hardcover)
1. Weight loss. 2. Reducing diets—Recipes. 3. Health. I. Title.
 RM222.2F845 2014
 613.2'5—dc23
                             2013047579

16 17 18 19   RRD(H)   10 9 8 7 6 5 4 3

I dedicate this book to all those who fight to save and improve our planet and the lives of its inhabitants. May our collective efforts bring a healthy future for our children and future generations.

Contents

The End of Dieting Pledge

We've been sold a false bill of goods.

Diets don't work, and they're terrible for our health.

Every diet is doomed to fail—whether it's counting calories or measuring portions or playing around with the ratio of fat, carbohydrate, and protein on your plate. Even if you do lose some weight, it usually returns within two years—and then some. In fact, the number of people who successfully lose weight through dieting and keep it off for the rest of their lives is fewer than two out of one hundred.[1] *Fewer than two out of one hundred.* That's less than 2 percent. That means that more than 98 percent of people who lose weight gain it back, which is often unhealthier than not losing it at all.

Constant fluctuations in weight and drastic changes to our diet are dangerous and likely to increase the risk of cardiovascular diseases.[2] In other words, we are literally killing ourselves in pursuit of a small waistline.

With its trendy, eat-this-not-that protocols and flavor-of-the-month celebrity weight-loss programs, the billion-dollar diet industry is hard at work making a mess of how we eat and how we think about food, while simultaneously selling temporary short-term fixes at the expense of our permanent long-term health.

And we've bought it, hook, line, and sinker.

As a result, our waistlines are thicker, and we're faced with an exploding worldwide epidemic of heart attack, stroke, diabetes, and cancer. You didn't fail those diets; the diets failed you.

We deserve better—better information, better food, better health. You deserve information that will work for you, so you never need to diet again.

Superior nutrition will transform your body and put an end to food addictions and cravings once and for all. My nutritarian way of eating satisfies all the dimensions of hunger. As you begin to eat healthful, nutrient-dense foods, such as vegetables, fruits, beans, nuts, and seeds, you flood your body with the vitamins, minerals, and phytochemicals that it so desperately needs. You will not only see immediate weight-loss benefits, your food preferences will also undergo a metamorphosis as you begin to crave health-supporting food instead of disease-causing food. The foods that once meant so much to you lose their appeal. And your bad emotionally based eating habits will start to disappear along with your waistline.

The nutritarian diet style makes it almost impossible to become overweight because you eat to satisfy true hunger, not addictive cravings. The foods you eat can be consumed in bountiful quantities because they are rich in nutrients, yet low in calories. You feel satisfied.

These next few sentences contain the secret to making this body transformation work every time, and it is my pledge to help you achieve the success you so deserve. In the beginning, let my brain call the shots, not yours. What you've done in the past hasn't worked out. We need to repair your brain first, and I'm going to show you how to do it. Don't make decisions about what to eat. Let me make those decisions for you. Get away from the stress of dieting and deciding what to eat and what not to eat almost every waking moment of the day. Don't judge how you're doing, or whether the foods you're eating are working. Just eat them. Within a week, the magic will begin.

The End of Dieting is the book and lifestyle you deserve. The dietary and nutritional advice presented in the following pages not only enables you to stop dieting for good, it prevents and reverses disease. And best of all, you can adjust it to meet your individual food preferences and individual dietary needs, which will allow you to reclaim, once and for all, your right to excellent health.

THE END OF DIETING

Introduction

Since its publication in 2003, *Eat to Live* has sold more than 1 million copies and has been translated into sixteen languages. It reached number one on the *New York Times* bestsellers list and has remained on the list for years, while hundreds, if not thousands, of other diet books have come and gone.

My goal for *Eat to Live* wasn't fame or fortune, however. When I sat down to write the book, I simply wanted to educate and motivate people to achieve superior health, whether they wanted to lose weight, feel great, or reverse a chronic disease. I had no idea the book would take off, or that it would resonate so deeply with people all around the world. It seemed everyone started using that phrase—eat to live—to describe the overwhelmingly successful eating style detailed in the book. And to this day, I receive a seemingly never-ending stream of e-mails and letters describing miraculous health changes, thanks to the book.

The secret behind *Eat to Live*'s popularity is simple: It didn't promise a quick fix. Unlike fad diets that promise easy and immediate results, *Eat to Live* laid out vital information about food and healthy eating that allowed readers to become experts in nutrition. The book essentially handed over to its readers the keys to successful weight management so that they were in control of their health destiny.

At the center of *Eat to Live* is a simple health equation, the core concept of my nutritarian program:

$$H = N / C$$
Health = Nutrients / Calories

Your health is predicted by your nutrient intake divided by your calorie intake.

I call this core concept the *nutrient density* of your diet. Food supplies us with both nutrients and calories (energy). All calories come from only three elements: carbohydrates, fats, and proteins. Nutrients, on the other hand, come from noncaloric food factors, namely, vitamins, minerals, fibers, and phytochemicals, literally chemical compounds that occur naturally in plants. These noncaloric nutrients are vitally important to your health. When the ratio of nutrients to calories is high, fat melts away, and health is restored. The more nutrient-dense food you consume, the more you'll be satisfied with fewer calories, and the less you'll crave fat and high-calorie foods.

A high-nutrient diet slows down the aging process, helps repair cells, reduces inflammation, and helps rid the body of toxins. High-nutrient, low-calorie foods contain a great deal of fiber and take up a lot of room in the stomach. As you consume a larger quantity of food, it satiates your hunger and blunts your appetite. Meeting the body's micronutrient needs also helps suppress food cravings and what I call "toxic hunger," which drives you to consume more calories than you require—usually in the form of processed foods, which can lead to cancer and heart disease, among many other ailments.

Witnessing how *Eat to Live* inspired so many people to change their diets not only reinforced my findings that high-nutrient diets produce good health, it offered a substantial, ongoing body of evidence proving that this approach works. Nothing shows the power of this way of eating more than hearing from people who apply this knowledge and live it every day in their own lives. Thousands of people lost dramatic amounts of weight without difficulty and never regained it. One reader named Scott weighed a staggering 500 pounds. Scott couldn't tie his own shoes. His breathing was labored, and he could walk only nine steps at a time. He was thirty-eight years old. A doctor told him that if he didn't undergo stomach reduction surgery, he would most likely die within six months. Scott spurned his doctor's advice and instead decided to change how he thought about food and his approach to eating by following my high-nutrient meal plan, which provided him with all the nutrients, protein, and vitamins he needed to achieve good health. Because he now eats for health, he can eat as much as he wants, fully ignoring the scale. Today, Scott weighs 180 pounds and loves to exercise—a big change from when he could hardly walk.

My patients routinely lose up to 20 pounds during the first six weeks of changing their eating habits. And that's just the beginning. More importantly, they typically recover from diseases such as allergies, asthma, acne, headaches, high blood pressure, diabetes, reflux esophagitis, lupus, kidney insufficiency, psoriasis, angina, cardiomyopathy, and multiple sclerosis—and they gradually get to eliminate their dependence on prescription drugs.

Though I have long studied and utilized high-nutrient eating as a medical prescription for the past twenty-five years, even I have to admit to being surprised by some of the phenomenal recoveries people have reported to me. Once, someone asked whether this micronutrient-rich approach could turn their hair back to brown from gray. "Of course not," I answered. But, sure enough, on my website forum two people commented that it had happened to them. I couldn't believe it. Similarly, one of my patients had hepatitis C before starting my eating style. I didn't think this high-nutrient eating style would cure his hepatitis infection and liver injury; however, after some time, his hepatitis C disappeared. I had to repeat the blood tests three times to believe it. Seeing such dramatic recoveries from what are conventionally considered irreversible diseases excited me, making me more adamant that this delicious way of eating can lead to medical transformations for millions of Americans.

The results and success stories are astounding. They come from people of different backgrounds, from different ages, and they all started their journeys for different reasons. Yet what they share in common is they are all now in excellent health.

For all of *Eat to Live*'s success, however, I quickly came to realize that science-based information about nutrition alone wasn't enough. With this information available to such a broad audience, why would so many people fail to recognize their need to protect their precious health and lose weight? Why would they be unable and unwilling to change? Why would they want to remain unhealthy? Why would they want to reject unassailable, scientific, and dramatically effective advice? I'll tell you why. Because of the overwhelming twin powers of food preference and food addiction.

Like the classic victim, we actually grow to love the things that kill us—in this case, unhealthy food. Unhealthy eating styles and food addictions have both taken control of our brains, and this addiction to certain foods is often as deadly as many other addictions.

The standard American diet (SAD) is killing us. Instead of providing us with our basic needs for good health, it has produced a nation where disease and chronic illness are considered to be inevitable and just another natural consequence of aging. Being overweight is the primary cause of type 2 diabetes; it accelerates atherosclerosis and death from heart disease. In a matter of years, excess body weight is projected to overtake smoking as the primary cause of death in the United States.[1] By the time most Americans reach the age of fifty, they are already hooked on prescription drugs, and almost half of Americans still die of heart attacks and strokes. You don't have to be one of them. Twenty-eight million Americans suffer from the crippling pain of osteoarthritis. You don't have to be one of them. Thirty-five million Americans suffer from chronic headaches. You don't have to be one of them. You simply don't have to be sick.

Today, 475 million adults around the world suffer from obesity. That's a 50 percent increase since 1980. At the same time, the number of overweight adults is quickly approaching 1 billion, and some 200 million school-age children are already overweight, which means nearly 1.7 billion people are either overweight or obese. *Nearly 1.7 billion people!*

In the United States alone, about two-thirds of Americans are overweight, according to the National Institutes of Health (NIH). But this doesn't tell the whole story. Both the NIH and the World Health Organization define an "overweight" person to have a body mass index (BMI) of 25. This means that a woman who is 5 feet 5 inches tall is considered a normal weight at 150 pounds, and a man who is 5 feet 10 inches tall is considered normal at 175 pounds. This man and woman may carry between 20 and 30 pounds of disease-causing fat around their waists, but they would still be considered healthy and fit by today's standards. This is simply not accurate to consider a person with that much fatty tissue normal or healthy. If you look at societies or groups of people who live longer than average, you'll find average BMIs between 18 and 22—nowhere near the American standard of 25. For example, the Okinawa Centenarian Study—which examined more than six hundred centenarians from Okinawa, Japan, over twenty-five years from the mid-1970s to 2001—found that the average BMI of the studied adults was 20.4. The Adventist Health Study—which studied Seventh-Day Adventists, who follow a largely vegan diet—found a similar result. This twelve-year prospective examination of thirty-four thousand middle-aged and elderly Adventists with no preexisting illnesses and no history of smoking, coronary heart disease, cancer, or stroke revealed a direct positive relation between a lower BMI and longevity. An Adventist with a BMI higher than 23 had a higher risk of premature death.

So what can we learn from these studies? According to the data, the *maximum* acceptable weight produces a BMI of around 22.5, not 25. This means that the recommended healthy weight for a 5-foot-10-inch adult male is between 130 and 160 pounds and for a 5-foot-5-inch adult female is 108 to 135 pounds. This is a big difference from the acceptable (not overweight) American BMI of 25, which allows 150 pounds for a woman and 175 pounds for a man.

On the basis of the Okinawan and Adventist standard BMI, about 85 percent of Americans are overweight, not the 66 percent according to the NIH. The average American is heavier and sicker than he or she even realizes. All because of the standard American diet. Hardly anyone can escape its destructive effects. Why else would 90 percent of everyone over the age of sixty-five be taking drugs to lower his or her blood pressure and/or cholesterol? The bottom line is this: If you eat American food, you will inevitably develop the diseases common in America, you will become overweight, and you will eventually develop high blood pressure and high cholesterol (the signs of blood vessel and heart disease), just like everybody else.

We now consider it normal to lose youthful vigor in our thirties, carry an extra 30 to 40 pounds, live with chronic illness in our late forties and fifties, and endure our final decades completely dependent on others. But this is *not* normal. This is the result of a lifelong pattern of unhealthy living and misguided information. Rather than dreading deterioration and a growing number of ailments and drugs as we approach old age, we should look forward to enjoying an active life well into our nineties. This may seem like an outrageous expectation because most of us spend a lifetime consuming an unhealthy diet. Even today, too many of us continue to miss the connection between what we eat and how we feel emotionally and physically. Nor can we figure out why it seems so difficult to stay at our young adult weight.

But it's not too late.

A high-nutrient diet will reduce your desire for high-calorie, low-nutrient foods. Within weeks, your taste buds will change, and you'll lose interest in the unhealthy foods you once thought you could never live without. You'll feel more satisfied eating fewer calories than you were eating before. The result is lasting health and permanent weight loss. So many of my readers have lost 100 pounds or more following my recommendations; they have lost that much within one year; and they have kept that weight off for years.

The End of Dieting goes a step beyond *Eat to Live*. Not only does it answer why eating healthfully often seems so difficult, it empowers you with the desire and ability to do so. In the following pages, I share the science and the solutions behind how to rid yourself for good of the food addictions sabotaging your health. I lay out an easy-to-follow eating program beginning with a fourteen-day series of easy-to-make, delicious meals that will gradually transform your food preferences, while simultaneously recalibrating your palate. I guide your food choices through the first part of the program, so you don't have to think or worry about what you're eating—you can simply eat tasty dishes made of fantastic health-supporting foods. In the second part of the program, I flood your body with nutrients to heal and detoxify it, using superfoods as a way to promote wellness and longevity. By completing and sticking to the program, your BMI will fall below 22.5 and stay there for the rest of your life.

A diet can only be considered successful if the food you eat supports longevity and protects you against heart disease, stroke, dementia, and cancer. This nutritarian diet style is the only dietary and nutritional program that guarantees dramatic weight loss without calorie counting. It is also the only dietary and nutritional program that teaches you how to protect against disease while simultaneously dramatically increasing your lifespan. Your risk of a heart attack and/or stroke will almost disappear, and your risk of cancer can plummet by more than 90 percent, while your life expectancy can increase by twenty years. Incredible claims, yes, but this is a reality with considerable scientific support. I have observed such results for more than twenty-five years.

Forget calories. The secret of living well is all about micronutrients. Eating healthfully and consuming the right assortment and amount of nutrients results in consistent, long-term health benefits. Getting healthy and maintaining a stable, healthy weight are achieved only by focusing on the nutritional quality of your food. Contrary to conventional thinking, it isn't *how much* you eat that determines your weight; it's what you eat.

Nutritional quality determines your mental, physical, and emotional health—from brain function and a heightened immune system to happiness and physical well-being. The main criterion you should consider when choosing what to eat is which foods are most favorable to your long-term survival. A diet style incorporating longevity-promoting foods allows you to try out all types of delicious recipes, which in turn allows you to keep up this new way of eating throughout the rest of your life. Any diet you adopt temporarily only results in temporary benefits, because eventually your body and your weight adjust back to the diet you will remain on long term.

Let me repeat that again: Anything you adopt temporarily only begets temporary results, and fluctuating your weight up and down is not lifespan favorable.

People often view diets as a belief system, picking the one that is most closely aligned with their dietary philosophy or food preferences. Then they often criticize any program that conflicts with these preferences. Real science, however, has no philosophy or predetermined agenda; it just flows inexorably from the preponderance of the evidence. Are you a scientific thinker? Are you willing to view the facts and let the chips fall with the evidence? Remember: Food preferences are learned and can be changed.

I have cared for more than ten thousand patients, most of whom set foot in my office unhappy, sick, and overweight. They had tried every dietary craze without success. After following my program, they discovered the superior health they always wanted and dropped the weight they always dreamed of losing. Even better, they kept it off. For the first time in their lives, they had an eating style that didn't leave them hungry or unsatisfied. Most importantly, they were able to stop taking their medications, which had become unnecessary.

Over the past three decades, I have reviewed more than twenty thousand scientific studies on human nutrition. This is why I can say with certainty that this is the place and now is the time to begin your health revival. I have seen the effects of this plan in action on thousands of patients with a wide range of diseases and health concerns, from migraines and allergies to heart disease and diabetes. The bottom line is, it works. Nutritional excellence is the most powerful way to discover permanent healthy weight loss, prevent and reverse disease, and put an end to some of today's most chronic degenerative illnesses.

The body is a self-healing machine when you supply it with an optimal nutritional environment, and the information presented in this book is the fastest and most effective way to create that environment. If you have high blood pressure, high cholesterol, diabetes, heart disease, indigestion, headache, asthma, fatigue, body aches, or pain—or if you want to prevent yourself from developing these chronic conditions—this is the plan for you. This new diet style can enable you to avoid angioplasty, bypass surgery, and other invasive procedures. If you aren't yet ill, it can make sure you never have heart attacks, strokes, or dementia in your later years. It can reduce and eventually eliminate your need for prescription drugs. In short, it can enable you to optimize your health and potentially save your life. And it can do all of this while increasing the pleasure you get from food.

Many of you have this book because you want to lose weight. I want to assure you that you *will* lose all the weight that you want, even if diets have failed you in the past. This is the most effective weight-loss plan ever, and the results are permanent, not temporary. Equally important is the protection from serious diseases in your future that this plan offers. The most effective healthcare is self-care. Drugs and doctors can't grant you excellent health and protect you from disease and suffering. Almost every doctor knows this. The nutritional excellence I describe in the following pages can prevent and even reverse most medical problems within three to six months. This is a bold claim, but the facts—backed up by scientific research—show that many of the tragedies we face in the modern world are the result of nutritional folly.

While weight loss is important, it is not our main goal. It is a pleasant and normal by-product on the road to the primary goal: great health. Superior health is marked by an exceptionally long and relatively disease-free lifespan, and countless studies reveal that people with superior health are slim. By teaching you how to achieve superior health, your ideal weight will naturally follow. You will understand the physical cravings that cause overeating, as well as the psychological factors that can help you change this pattern of consumption. Applying the information in this book to your life will help you create new, healthy behaviors that will eventually become effortless. You will finally be in control of your own health destiny.

This plan does not include counting calories, measuring portion sizes, or weighing. It doesn't rely on gimmicks or fads. You can stop looking for that magic solution, because there is no magic solution. No red berry ketones. No green coffee beans. No purple tulip nectar or black salt from the white cliffs of Dover. In fact, we almost always later discover that the product that gave us hope was merely hype and that looking for a quick fix causes harm. When a supplement or medication doesn't meet your nutritive needs, it is typically toxic and can enhance the damage caused by a toxic diet.

In Their Own Words

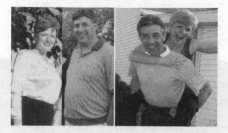

Cassie and Dave, alarmed by increasing symptoms associated with poor health and aging, made a decision to Eat to Live. Hoping for many positive changes for themselves, they were pleasantly surprised by the added benefits for the rest of the family.

BEFORE: 162 pounds (Cassie) and 250 pounds (Dave)

AFTER: 111 pounds (Cassie) and 145 pounds (Dave)

My husband, Dave, and I have been happily married for twenty-five years. We have four children, all in their twenties, and a young grandson. We were only in our late forties, yet we felt very old, unhealthy, tired, and frustrated. We experienced brain fog and lack of energy daily, constant sinus infections, migraines, back pain, indigestion, eczema, severe mood swings, and agonizing cravings and food addictions. Our toxic diet and sedentary lifestyle were taking their toll.

One transformative day we discovered Dr. Fuhrman's teachings. We immediately threw out all our processed foods and eliminated meat, dairy, oil, salt, and sweeteners from our diet. *Eat to Live* became our daily manual. It provided us with the knowledge that we needed to succeed. Our motivation wasn't weight driven; rather, it was driven by a deep passion to get healthy and change our lives for the better.

Our physical and mental transformations have been amazing! After thirty-five years, Dave even finally quit coffee and cigarettes. He and I now walk, run, or hike at least twenty to twenty-five miles a week and incorporate cardio and calorie-burning exercises into our daily routine. We both feel great.

Our transformation and passionate commitment to our new nutritarian diet style have allowed our new lifestyle to positively affect our children as well. They have also incorporated our food choices into their diets and, as a result, have experienced significant weight loss and overall health improvements.

The one truth that we have learned with our nutritarian lifestyle is that we all have the power to take control of our own health destiny—it's in each one of us!

Nor do you have to become a vegan or vegetarian to prevent a heart attack and reduce the risk of cancer. You just have to incorporate life-enhancing, delicious, and natural plant foods and significantly cut back on animal products. Eat as much food as you want, and, over a short time, you'll be more than satisfied with the fewer number of calories you're consuming.

This is a diet style that you will learn to enjoy forever. The goal is for the information to change you in a natural fashion, so this style becomes your preferred way of eating. To accomplish this, I'll present scientific, logical information that explains the connection between food and your health. By incorporating this information into your life and using the included meal plans and delicious recipes, you'll shed pounds consistently and almost miraculously—the natural side effect of eating so healthfully. You will also discover an amazing new array of different flavors and foods that will soon become your preferred way to eat.

Can any other program produce these results and support the claims with real science? Can another program present thousands of weight-loss and disease-reversal successes from people who have already adopted it, lost their excess weight, and kept it off over many years? Can any other program stand the test of time and scrutiny of the scientific community for effectiveness and consistency with established and emerging science? Of course not, and that grants you a supportive community of many thousands of people anxious to share their success, offer tips, and camaraderie and support you along your path to wellness. You can see how others can be so helpful by reading some of these people's stories, in their own words, throughout this book.

I promise you, through this diet style, you can retain your youthful vigor and health. You can prevent heart attacks, strokes, dementia, and even cancer. You will literally disease-proof your body—all while losing weight. You'll come to understand the key principles of the science of health, nutrition, and weight loss. And, as a result, you'll gain a simple and effective strategy to achieve—and maintain—a favorable weight without dieting for the rest of your life, freeing you forever from a merry-go-round of endless, tedious discussions about dieting strategies.

The cases incorporated into this book are submissions from people in their own words, chosen, out of hundreds submitted, because they exemplify the experience of many and share a learning point that can benefit you on your quest to a happy and fulfilled life. They have agreed to use their actual names because they are enthusiastic and committed to having a positive effect on the lives of others. What they have learned has freed them from dieting—for the rest of their lives. They, and I, hope you will be inspired to do the same.

Welcome to the end of dieting.

IN THEIR OWN WORDS

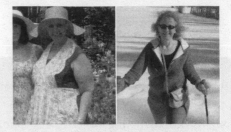

Kathleen spent her life on the dieting merry-go-round as the result of food addiction and cravings. Her dysfunctional relationship with food controlled her life, until she took back her power.

BEFORE: 228 pounds

AFTER: 163 pounds (so far)

Food was the perfect friend. This friend never, ever let me down. If I was sad, food was there for me. If I wanted to celebrate, my "friend" lifted me up and celebrated with me. If I was bored, food filled my time. If life was too painful to contemplate, my friend distracted me, easing my pain. Truly, food felt like the best friend I'd ever had.

The standard American diet brought me solace, comfort, celebration. It was always present when I was lonely. However, it also brought me pain and despair because this relationship caused me to gain an enormous amount of weight. It exacerbated a genetic condition, causing me to end up with such severe osteoarthritis that I had to have a total knee replacement. I was only forty-seven years old. The standard American diet, and my addiction to food, chipped away at my self-esteem and self-care.

Clearly, the sensible thing to do was to end this unhealthy relationship. But, as with all dysfunctional relationships, ending it also meant giving up the good parts that I desperately wanted. How does one reconcile that? I suspect that the answer to this question is deeply personal and different for each of us. For me, it took watching my dad slowly die, a victim of the standard American diet. I remember visiting my dad in the ICU after he'd pulled through yet another crisis and suggesting to him that he could improve his health by improving his diet. He shook his head and said, "Kathleen, I can't give up my food." I'll never forget his words as he sat in his hospital bed under the harsh fluorescent lights with the sound of monitors beeping in the background. He had just nearly died, and yet he couldn't give up his unhealthy foods. Wow. That's addiction for you. Not only did I miss him terribly when he passed, but I also saw my own future. My addiction to the standard American diet was no less powerful than my dad's, and I was terrified.

I worked with Dr. Fuhrman's food addiction counselor, who helped me recognize my dysfunctional relationship with food. I realized that my addiction to food was no different from an addiction to drugs or alcohol. Aren't we so very fortunate that our addiction is socially sanctioned and it takes place in clean church halls, restaurants, and our very own kitchens? Aren't we lucky that we don't have to hide in dirty alleys to get our fixes? And isn't it incredibly tragic that we have the same exact sort of dopamine-craving, soul-crushing, health-destroying compulsion that the drug addict has?

I also learned that if you're running with a crowd that causes you trouble, you end up making poor decisions. This crowd doesn't respect you. It hurts you. You have to cut those friends loose no matter what positive aspects the relationship brings to you. For me, unhealthy food was my dysfunctional "gang."

As so often happens when you remove dysfunctional relationships from your life, you open up space to form new, healthy connections. I now have gorgeous, fresh, crisp vegetables as friends. I have decadently sweet, juicy fruit. I have happy belly-filling beans, hearty whole grains, and luscious nuts and seeds. My new friends nourish me and never hurt me the way the standard American diet always did. Now that I have a much healthier relationship with food, I'm 60 pounds lighter and I'm still losing weight.

Breaking free of food addiction is difficult, but once you have the knowledge provided by Dr. Fuhrman's research and writings, you can never un-know it. Once you've had the experience of living in a truly nourished body, you can never again tolerate the toxic feelings that come from toxic food. Once you start to become active, you can never tolerate stagnation again. Once you learn to listen to your own body, you'll always hear its wisdom.

Part
ONE

Toxic Hunger

We have a nation of overweight and sickly people, with health care costs out of control. We have people suffering from easily preventable diseases all around us. Why isn't everyone recognizing that a radical change in our nation's diet is needed to fix this? Why are we so confused about nutrition? The evidence of this crisis is all around us, but this state of affairs is not a coincidence. The traditional food pyramid, once the cornerstone of the U.S. Department of Agriculture (USDA), and the standard American diet (SAD) are both responsible for our poor health and our poor information.

Influenced by social, business, and political concerns—rather than pure nutritional science—the food pyramid recommended massive amounts of foods that were high in calories and generally low in nutrients, such as white bread, oils, and chicken. The current government plate is an improvement over the past pronouncements, but still leaves much to be desired, and the diet style of Americans has not changed for the better. The majority of calories in the American diet still come from refined, processed foods and fast foods. Fifty-five percent of calories now come from processed foods and 30 percent from animal products, both of which are dangerously lacking in antioxidants and phytochemicals, two essential life-protecting and life-saving classes of nutrients. There's no way around it. A diet centered on milk, cheese, pasta, bread, fried foods, and sugar-filled snacks and drinks leads to obesity, cancer, heart disease, diabetes, and autoimmune illnesses.

We're eating ourselves to death.

Simply put, the SAD is toxic. There is no better word to describe it. It causes disease and leads to compulsive eating. It's terrible for us, and terribly addictive. Our standard diet of foods high in fat, sugar, and salt are physically addictive, which makes it impossible for most people to reduce portion sizes, cut back on calories, count points, or follow other typical dieting strategies.

Unhealthy Food Is Powerfully Addicting

Most researchers believe that 5 to 10 percent of the U.S. population is addicted to food. Not me. I believe that 60 to 80 percent of the population suffers from food addiction—and this is true whether someone is eating processed food, a low-nutrient diet, or even a high-protein diet based on animal products. People who are overweight struggle with sweets, fried foods, chips, and fatty meats in exactly the same way smokers and drug addicts struggle with cigarettes and cocaine.

If you're overweight, chances are you're a food addict. You eat because you physically feel the need for food, not because your body has any biological need for additional calories.

Addiction is a physical and psychological dependence on a substance or behavior. Initially, the substance or behavior satisfies a person, but it quickly turns to compulsion when he or she needs more, just to avoid the discomfort or pain that follows. Food addiction is complex and involves the stimulation of the digestive apparatus, which results in the release of bile, enzymes, and hormones and removes waste from the liver, kidney, and bloodstream. It also intimately involves dopamine in the brain. A primary neurotransmitter, dopamine regulates, among other things, motivation and feelings of pleasure. Regardless of the addiction, the brain reacts in the same way. Concentrated calories like sugar and oil, for instance, produce within food addicts a surge in dopamine levels similar to the levels found in people who abuse illegal drugs.

Investigators from Boston Children's Hospital in Massachusetts recently found that a meal high in refined carbohydrates produced brain effects consistent with those of drug addiction.[1] Every single subject showed intense activation in the nucleus accumbens, the area of the brain related to addiction.

The brain is literally wired to ensure that we repeat behaviors that make us feel good by associating them with the sweet release of dopamine and specific brain patterning. The brain records a pleasurable action as a beneficial pattern that needs to be remembered and repeated automatically. The smoker lights up a cigarette, for instance, and the food addict opens a bag of potato chips without hesitation or any consideration of the long-term risks.

And just as the smoker becomes tolerant to nicotine, the overeater becomes tolerant to sugar and salt and fat, reducing the amount of pleasure derived from eating high-caloric foods. A recent study published in *Nature Neuroscience* showed that drug addiction and compulsive eating desensitize brain reward circuits.[2] This means that to feel the pleasure of drugs or the pleasure of eating, we need more and more. In the brain, eating behavior is driven by pleasure and reward signals, and the brain now needs lots of stimulation (concentrated food that is highly sweetened and flavored) or lots of eating to maintain those signal levels. Anything less results in physical and emotional discomfort.

I have never really thought of it as food addiction, but reading what you have said, I see that my father died from food addiction. He was a physician and was diagnosed with type 2 diabetes when he was thirty-seven. After years of using medications (eleven of them) to treat his symptoms while buying candy and pastries in bulk, he died at the ripe age of sixty-four. I now see that this was addictive behavior because he knew that changing his diet would make his symptoms go away. He knew what the consequences of his behavior would be and yet he kept gorging on unhealthy food for twenty-five years. Twenty-five years of hospital stays and all sorts of nasty diabetic side effects. He was not a dummy, yet he engaged in this irrational behavior.

Angela Biggar

Most overweight people understand that being overweight is bad for their health. Their friends and family and even their doctors may have advised them to lose weight, but they can't. They have tried diet after diet but simply can't stick to them. Why does this happen? Why can't they just stop eating?

The answer is TOXIC HUNGER.

When we eat primarily foods high in calories, without incorporating sufficient amounts of protective nutrients into our diets, our cells become congested with waste products such as free radicals and advanced glycation end products (AGEs), collectively known as *oxidative stress*. Oxidative stress can lead to inflammation, cell damage, and premature cell death. More often than not, it is accompanied by a buildup of toxic metabolites that can create physical symptoms of withdrawal between meals. I call these withdrawal symptoms *toxic hunger.*

If you feel any of the following symptoms, you're experiencing toxic hunger.

Weakness

Fatigue

Shakiness

Headache

Stomach fluttering or cramping

AM I A FOOD ADDICT? TEST YOURSELF.

1. If I don't eat regularly, I feel fatigued or irritable.	Yes or No
2. I think about eating certain foods almost all the time.	Yes or No
3. I feel sluggish or uncomfortable after eating.	Yes or No
4. Eating poorly is interfering with my health.	Yes or No
5. I'm overweight, but I continue to overeat.	Yes or No
6. When I start eating sweets, I don't want to stop.	Yes or No

7. I have tried to diet to lose weight, but failed and given up.   Yes or No

8. I prefer restaurants with all-you-can-eat buffets.   Yes or No

9. I have physical withdrawal symptoms.   Yes or No

10. I sneak food when others aren't around or looking.   Yes or No

11. I store food or hide food from my family.   Yes or No

12. I eat more even though I'm no longer hungry.   Yes or No

13. My eating habits cause me distress.   Yes or No

14. My eating habits are causing me social and family difficulties.   Yes or No

15. I eat almost continuously all day long.   Yes or No

One "yes" answer makes you a suspected food addict. Two or more "yes" answers confirm your addiction to food.

Discomfort after stopping an addictive substance is called *withdrawal,* and it is significant because it represents detoxification or a biochemical healing after a substance is withdrawn. It's nearly impossible to cleanse the body of a harmful substance without experiencing discomfort. Detoxification is enhanced when digestion ceases. So when digestion is finished, people often feel queasy, tired, or headachy and most often believe that these minor discomforts are actual feelings of hunger. Eating something restarts digestion and shuts down the detoxification process, which helps make the bad feelings go away. Let me explain.

There are two phases of the digestive cycle, the anabolic and catabolic. During the anabolic, or building, phase, you eat, chew, digest, and absorb nutrients, which slows or halts the active process of detoxification that occurs most efficiently when the body's not actively digesting food. When digestion stops, the body enters its catabolic phase, and detoxification immediately starts to rev up. As a result, people experience detox symptoms, which they interpret as hunger. They just *have* to eat again, they think, even though their body is already overfilled with calories. They can either eat frequently so their body doesn't enter the catabolic phase for any sustained time, or they can eat calorically dense meals and animal products to keep the digestion (anabolic) process active until it's time to eat again.

The distinction between real hunger and toxic hunger is crucial. Unlike true hunger, which appears when the body has burned through most of the stored calories from the previous meal and is now ready to be refueled, toxic hunger occurs when the body starts to get rid of these dangerous toxins. We immediately feel discomfort, which makes us think we need to eat or drink a high-caloric load for relief. This drives overeating behavior and strongly increases your desire to consume more calories than the body requires.

> I am not asking you to diet. I'm asking you to change your fundamental beliefs about food.

The more you search for quick relief, however, the more you inhibit the detoxification, or healing, process. Uncomfortable sensations are very often the signals that repair is under way and the removal of toxins is occurring. We mistake these symptoms for actual hunger and, as a result, mistakenly eat too often and too much to lessen them, which causes us to pack on the pounds, make ourselves sick, and, in the process, perpetuate the vicious cycle of addiction.

Quitting a bad habit initially makes you feel worse, not better. When people start a healthy diet, for instance, the first three to five days are usually the most uncomfortable. This is precisely why all diets fail. No matter the diet, they all try to get people to eat less, and eating less is too uncomfortable physically and emotionally. The only way to comfortably eat less is to help the body desire less food, which requires us to get rid of the toxic hunger. Micronutrient adequacy is needed to prevent the buildup of toxins in cells, a primary cause of toxic hunger. In order to gravitate comfortably toward a more favorable weight, our diet has to be healthier and more micronutrient complete.

In Their Own Words

Heather doesn't worry about the scale anymore. She eats what she wants and is far healthier and headache-free.

BEFORE: 201 pounds

AFTER: 125 pounds

I'm a thirty-eight-year-old wife and mother of three. For as long as I can remember, I've suffered from horrible, debilitating migraines. I couldn't sleep. I was exhausted all the time. I didn't have the energy to get up and play with my son and would nod off while driving (yikes!). I suffered from terrible seasonal allergies and had an unexplained facial rash that didn't go away for months. I also had mood swings, although my family tells me that I was just plain grumpy. I started taking an antidepressant for anxiety.

I tried to start my own plan to regain my health. I ordered a juicer and juiced for about four weeks. Although I felt great, I knew this wasn't a way I could live long term. I considered this time as just a detox for my body in preparation for what was yet to come.

Inspired to learn more, I did some research and found Dr. Fuhrman. I discovered his books, bought one, and read it in one day. This book is now marked up like my Bible.

I used to be a food label reader (you can see where that got me), but I've since learned that I was looking for the wrong things—carbs and protein, for example, which are emphasized in the standard American diet. I don't buy anything processed or packaged, so labels hardly matter to me anymore. However, when I buy canned goods, such as beans or tomato sauce, I buy organic and am always vigilant about the amount of salt and sugar they contain. I will NEVER eat the other way again, EVER.

Since becoming a nutritarian I've lost weight, but more importantly, I feel FANTASTIC! I haven't had a cold in over a year. I no longer suffer from migraines or headaches. I have energy. I sleep well. I stopped taking antidepressants, and I no longer suffer from anxiety. I feel GREAT all the time!

What you choose to eat is an opportunity to control how your brain functions. It is an opportunity to control your emotional and physical well-being and to control your later-life health. The key is to get all parts of your brain to agree to eat healthfully, because part of you may not want to go along. Once you understand how an unhealthful diet style can take over the brain, you can earn back your health and discover an ideal weight.

Beat the Brain at Its Own Game

So how and where do you start? You may have a New Year's resolution or want to look great in that bathing suit for the Fourth of July. But it doesn't work that way. It's not about will power. There are no shortcuts. Addictions don't respond to easy answers. You can't "just say no."

The first step to resolving food addiction is to eat lots of micronutrient-rich produce, which will crowd out the junk food and, over time, lessen toxic hunger signals and eventually eliminate your craving for junk. Fill your stomach with foods that have a high-nutrient, low-calorie density—foods such as raw vegetables, fruits, beans, onions, and mushrooms, which help you beat your addiction and lose weight. These fill up your stomach so much that you won't feel like eating the concentrated calories found in addictive foods.

Ice cream is addictive, for instance. A peach is not. A peach won't make you want to eat a dozen of them in a druglike binge. With its heavy concentration of sugar and fat, ice cream will light up a primitive part of your brain that persuades you to give up control, just as cocaine persuades coke addicts to let their lives spin out of control.

The most effective way to lose weight safely is to give up the goal of losing weight in favor of preventing disease and living pain free later in life. You'll now eat more of the disease-fighting foods and fewer or none of the disease-causing foods. And by eating a high-grade nutritarian diet, you'll cycle through the detox phase so quickly that you'll be feeling fine in just a few days. Toxic hunger will fade away, and you won't be driven to eat all the time.

To Beat Food Addiction, You Also Have to Beat Emotional Eating

Toxic hunger keeps us in a spiral of bad choices and leads to food addiction. But there is an additional obstacle that many of us need to overcome: emotional eating. Emotional eating is the other side of the biological basis of food addiction. When people turn to food to relieve their stress, they're really just falling back on bad habits, reaching for the foods they've always eaten. When people continue to eat foods that they know aren't good for them, this too is the result of an emotional need. We have all experienced choosing a short-term calorie load of fat, sugar, or carbs to avoid the negative emotions after a tough day. To upend emotional eating, we have to change our mind-set. We must break the bad habits we have formed and discover the necessary self-esteem to continue to make good, healthy choices every day.

Habits, it turns out, are the same in low- and high-pressure situations. In good times or bad, people simply do what they've always done, defaulting to their regular habits—whether it's eating, smoking, or biting their nails. So how do you break a bad habit? By developing good habits.

Yes, it takes a conscious, concerted effort to break old habits. It takes time to develop good habits. It takes time to retrain your taste buds. It takes time to heal the body and repair the damage. It takes time to feel true hunger rather than toxic hunger. But, trust me, it's worth it.

Here's the secret, though, about learning to eat well. You can't develop good eating habits without simultaneously developing good emotional habits. The two go hand in hand. Emotional eating is when you eat for comfort during moments of great difficulty or high stress. Sweets and other disease-causing foods take you to a place of bliss. To get off the dieting merry-go-round once and for all, you have to build up your self-esteem, because the happier and healthier you feel, the less likely you are to resort to food, drugs, or alcohol to cope.

Feeling good about yourself is an active process. It involves *doing*. For many people, self-esteem stems from exercise. For others, it comes with a job well done. For some, it's a product of helping others or developing a new skill. Losing weight and finding health can be a powerful boost to your self-confidence and self-esteem, but they occur only once you start to strengthen every aspect of your life. Focus on that before focusing on the numbers on your scale.

Just as junk food weakens the brain, self-doubt weakens the will. The combination of healthy eating and healthy emotional habits can heal both.[3] This involves changing behaviors that will strengthen your emotional health and change the emphasis of your life—from how you approach food to how you interact with people. Using food as an emotional crutch prevents you from learning proper coping skills and developing vital social skills necessary to successfully navigate life. When you are under stress and need comforting, try talking to someone. A connection to others, coupled with a felt responsibility for others, translates into a sense of purpose and self-worth, which usually results in better health. A meta-analysis of 148 studies on the correlation between strong relationships and good health indicated a 50 percent increase in the likelihood of survival for the more than three hundred thousand participants who enjoyed strong social relationships. This finding remained consistent across age, sex, health status, cause of death, and follow-up period.[4] The message here is that working on building friendships and helping others doesn't merely make you healthier and extend your life; it is also an effective strategy for resolving food addiction.

Marriage On the Rocks, High Blood Pressure, and Prediabetes

A perfect example is Jill Harrington, a patient of mine. Jill was over-weight, unhappy, and disappointed in her marriage. She complained about her aloof husband and felt trapped in the relationship. She considered divorce, but couldn't afford one. Her husband, Tim, ate poorly and drank alcohol almost every night. Jill was trying to follow my program but found it difficult, especially with the stress of her marriage. Tim hardly ever paid attention to her.

Jill and Tim were essentially living together as roommates; there was no romance in their marriage. I wanted to help Jill lose weight and find happiness, but I knew the trouble in her marriage was one of the biggest obstacles to her success. Therefore, I worked on a strategy with her to help improve her marriage so she could focus her energy on eating better. This was an essential first step in improving her health and happiness. Instead of placing demands on Tim, for instance, she started to thank him for the small things he always did for her. At the same time, she came up with a few small things she could do for him. We talked at length about Tim and his many good points, as well as all the reasons she still loved him. I spent some time with her bringing out Tim's good points and reasons she loved him over the years. I told her that she should be proud of her ability to care for, support, and show her love for him unconditionally.

Jill immediately started feeling better about herself, living with more confidence, and Tim, to his credit, responded in kind. He was kinder and more thoughtful too. Eventually, they were both more af-fectionate toward one another, emotionally and physically. Their mar-riage was moving in a better direction. As a result, Jill gave up her disappointment in Tim and finally agreed that their marital problems weren't merely his fault. She acknowledged her role in them as well. In time, they rekindled a healthy marital relationship.

As that part of her life improved, Jill's diet and health simultaneously improved. Instead of eating emotionally, she ate nutritarian meals and started to feel in control of her life and her food choices. She finally was able to look better and feel better and successfully stop taking her medications. She was on her way to better health.

Like Jill, your emotional health depends on your feeling good about yourself—not because you tell yourself you love yourself or because someone else does, but rather because of your positive actions. To assure success, you need a legitimate reason to love yourself for your ability to appreciate the value, importance, goodness, and beauty around you. Not by trying to impress, but rather by trying to feel. Not by trying to make yourself look good, but rather by trying to appreciate how much beauty is in others. How much you are loved isn't the most important thing. A better measurement of emotional strength is your capacity to emote and feel love for others.

The Three Habits of Health

The way you take care of yourself is just as crucial a determinant of your future happiness as your savings account. Many people invest in their financial future, but they never consider their health future. A large nest egg is of no use to you if you're not there to spend it!

As you plan for your health future, you must consider the three important components that pay the biggest dividends: nutrition, exercise, and positive mind-set.

- Nutrition: Make every calorie count as you strive for lifelong health. Strive only to eat foods that are rich in nutrients and low in calories—and remember my health equation, H (Health) = N (Nutrition) / C (Calories).

- Exercise: Exercise regularly. Make it a part of your daily routine. A gym membership is nice, but there are plenty of other opportunities to work out your body over the course of an average day. Take the stairs, for instance, instead of the elevator. Walk or ride a bike instead of drive. Take frequent exercise breaks and do something active for just three to five minutes, then go back to work.

• Positive mind-set: A healthy mind-set is a prerequisite for a healthy lifestyle. The best way to develop one is to be optimistic and surround yourself with people who engage in and support your health. Show people you care about them with your actions, not just with words. A positive mind-set results from your goodwill to others. It is like putting deposits in your lifespan account.

These are the three essential habits of health. The more you practice them, the more routine they become. You won't want to act any other way.

Many people—healthy and unhealthy people alike—are often obsessed with food. Eating the right foods will make you incredibly healthy, but avoid obsessions even with healthful foods because they are often indicators of compulsions and other emotional and psychological issues. Striking a balance between eating and not eating is the quickest way to eliminate this obsession and live a fully balanced life where people, food, and exercise are all in the right place. The key to finding food's place in this delicate balance is by practicing the habits of health until they all become a natural part of your life. Balancing your diet style for optimal health is part of, and most natural and effective when it is connected to, balancing your life between exercise, rest, sleep, recreation, work, family, friends, and intellectual pursuits.

Addictions make attempts at dietary modifications more difficult, but it only takes a few seconds of decision-making to win the battle and say an emphatic "no" to your destructive compulsions and a resounding "yes" to the three habits of health. Throughout my career, I have observed thousands of people in whom these positive changes have resulted in tremendous benefits. Sure, there are always some temporary moments of discomfort as the body eliminates toxins and restores its cells to a more youthful, decongested state. This is perfectly normal, however. Learning to cope is a small price to pay for better health. Never underestimate the human body's powerful capacity for self-healing when superior nutrition takes the place of dietary and emotional distress.

Mild cravings will always come and go. From time to time, you may still want to eat unhealthy food or eat when you're not truly hungry. But remember: You always have a choice. Modern foods—the products of a manipulative, profit-driven food industry—are designed to seduce your taste buds. They entice us to eat even when we're not truly hungry, and the intense, artificial flavors cause us to enjoy natural flavors less. Our taste buds get all out of whack, and we become captives of these heightened flavors. Fortunately, by eating a high-nutrient diet, your cravings lessen and your sensory abilities return—like never before.

Realizing your impediments and gaining knowledge about great health are important steps toward lifelong health. But you also have to put into practice and repeat the three habits of health—nutrition, exercise, and positive mind-set—over and over again until they become part of you. Repetition breeds positive action. The more you eat healthful meals, and the more days you link together nutrition, exercise, and a positive mind-set, the more your brain will respond to them—and the more you'll come to prefer eating healthfully.

Cultivating a desire for optimal health will help in this process. Eat right, and your taste buds will line up with this desire, and your behaviors will work in concert with your new beliefs. Before you know it, you won't even want artificially flavored or heavily seasoned foods. You'll crave healthy, naturally flavored foods.

It's never easy to develop new habits, and there's no such thing as a shortcut to developing them. However, if you're motivated to persevere and keep trying, the change soon becomes considerably easier. Feeling better and losing weight are great motivators. Don't give up. The only way to fail is to stop trying.

IN THEIR OWN WORDS

Ronna didn't need to lose a significant amount of weight, but her food cravings and addictions were ruling her life—until she embraced a nutritarian lifestyle.

BEFORE: 146 pounds

AFTER: 116 pounds

My head was once filled with a myriad of nutrition theories. Self-help books and fad diets dictated my rules for weight loss. I was only concerned with finding the right diet program for a "miraculous" weight loss. To me, increasing vitamins and minerals meant consuming supplements and fortified foods, such as orange juice and cereals. Having salad or a side of some vegetable was my version of observing the food pyramid. I avoided junk food and tried to eat less—but it did not work.

At age eleven, I was diagnosed with an underactive thyroid, which meant I could only lose weight through extreme calorie restriction and/or excessive physical activity. I was a classic yo-yo dieter. I could never stay away from sugar for very long. I became addicted to sweets and felt I needed to diet like crazy to compensate.

After attending one of Dr. Fuhrman's Health Immersion programs, however, I started reading his books, which dramatically shifted my perspective on many health-related matters. Before the immersion, I fed my desires daily—coffee with cream, a little wine and cheese, several bites of a gluten-free ice-cream sandwich and a few "healthy snacks," which I thought I needed every few hours.

My erroneous beliefs didn't end there. I had self-diagnosed myself as hypoglycemic, but I wasn't. I was just going through withdrawals from my toxic diet. I also believed that my metabolism would slow down with age and that my hypothyroid disease was working against me, both of which proved to be myths.

Becoming a nutritarian changed my life. I don't just look different; I think and live differently. I have shed 30 pounds from my 5-foot-2-inch frame. My energy battery is always fully charged, and I'm no longer a slave to addictive eating habits. I'm happier and think more clearly. I feel a sense of balance, ease in movement, and enhanced self-confidence. And, most importantly, my cravings and the constant "noise" in my head related to food, body weight, and self-image are completely gone.

CHAPTER TWO

Diet Myths
Exposed

In a 1954 study published in the *Journal of Abnormal Psychology,* researchers asked Princeton and Dartmouth college students to watch a football game between the two schools and pay attention to penalties. Not surprisingly, the Princeton students reported twice as many violations by the Dartmouth team as the students from Dartmouth did. Likewise, a more recent study asked people to identify whether highly credentialed and respected scientists were credible experts on global warming, nuclear waste, and gun control. Subjects favored the scientists whose conclusions matched their own values; the facts or their expertise were irrelevant.

This behavior, called *selective perception,* happens when rational and intelligent people distort facts by seeing them through the lens of their personal perceptions and preferences. They wind up with views that are incorrect and out of whack with reality. Selective perception affects our beliefs so much that it can stand in the way of scientific communication, which helps explain the continued popularity of wildly outrageous, dangerous, and scientifically unsound diets.[1]

Like any other person, health writers and medical authorities approach their subjects with inherent biases, agendas, and egos, all of which color their findings and influence how they package information. Everywhere I look, board-certified doctors and celebrity nutritionists are promoting falsehoods, while shelling out improper advice about food and nutrition. When these so-called experts continue to hold on to their biases about nutrition despite the mounting scientific evidence against them, everybody loses.

What we hear today about nutrition and dieting is, at best, confusing. Almost every article or television show on the topic hypes some magic food, supplement, metabolism booster, fasting protocol, or fat-carbohydrate-protein ratio that can instantly solve all of our weight problems. Research articles continue to test diets that are low in fat, high in fat, low in carbohydrates, or high in carbohydrates, and the media continue to report on them as though they were exciting new breakthroughs.

But trying to micromanage carbohydrate, fat, or protein has never been shown to substantially increase health and longevity. This sort of restrictive dieting only encourages drastic fluctuations in caloric intake, which, as we already learned, result in only temporary changes in body weight.

Meanwhile, study after study shows that diets that fail to address nutritional quality fail to make any real dent in weight loss or other health parameters.[2] A magic ratio of fat, carbohydrate, and protein that will lead you to your ideal weight and superior health doesn't exist. Weight loss and superior health are the products of substantive changes in the nutritional quality of the food you eat. Whatever ratio of fat, protein, and carbohydrate you eat doesn't matter (within reason, of course). It is predominantly the nutritional quality and healthfulness of those carbs, fats, and proteins that determine your health.

Who Do You Believe?

In the field of nutritional science, getting the science right is critically important because even small errors of perception or interpretation can result in bad health—and even the loss of human life. To counter this, nutritionists must come to a consensus about the ideal way to eat. If we simply accepted some basic irrefutable truths about nutrition and health, rather than looking for the newest fad diet, our country wouldn't be mired in a terrifying health and obesity pandemic.

The three irrefutable facts about health and foods are these:

1. Vegetables, beans, seeds, fruits, and nuts are good for you.

2. Excessive amounts of meat or animal products cause disease.

3. Eliminating refined carbohydrates will aid in sustainable weight loss and overall health.

A diet style composed of the healthiest foods is the healthiest. As ridiculously obvious as this sounds, a mystifying majority of us still struggle to accept this simple fact: For a diet style to be truly healthful, it absolutely must contain large amounts of vegetables. The scientific literature backing this up is unimpeachable.

And yet, we all continue to get distracted by the latest fad diets—largely because the standard American diet is so markedly dangerous that even the most scientifically suspect diet looks better in comparison. For instance, when you read or hear about how the Mediterranean diet reduces your chances of heart disease and cardiac arrest by 25 percent, it looks good in relation to the SAD, which is responsible for 1.5 million heart attacks each year in the United States. I don't know about you, but a 25 percent reduction in the risk of heart disease doesn't excite me. I want it reduced by 100 percent.[3] This is especially relevant since any diet that still allows so many cardiovascular deaths, as today's Mediterranean diet, should not be held in high esteem, but instead considered dangerous.

Judging the merits of a mediocre diet plan against a terrible one doesn't improve your health. Comparing the Mediterranean diet to the SAD and demonstrating benefits is like buying a car by comparing it to a junkyard wreck. There are hundreds of popular diets out there. The famous DASH diet. The Weight Watchers diet. The Biggest Loser diet. The TLC diet. The Flat Belly diet. The Jenny Craig diet. Not to mention the crash diets and fasting protocols that are doomed to fail. I could go on and on and evaluate each one, but I won't waste my time or yours. Instead, I'll break down five specific diets—the standard American diet, the Paleo diet, the Mediterranean diet, the Wheat Belly diet, and low-fat veganism. These five approaches, which the majority of Americans consider to be healthy, are in truth potentially harmful and keep you trapped in the vicious cycle of toxic hunger and overeating. I'll then measure each one against a nutritarian approach to eating to demonstrate how and why we can break free from this cycle once and for all.

The Standard American Diet: It's to Die For

Some people like to think that there's nothing wrong with the SAD, for them it's perfect. The only thing perfect about the SAD is that it's perfectly designed to kill us off.

The SAD is centered on chicken, red meat, cheese, and other animal products, sweets, and processed grains, particularly wheat. Even worse, the typical person eating this way consumes a tremendous amount of extracted vegetable oil. Not only does oil supply lots of empty calories, it also contains a suspected carcinogen—called 3-MCPD, or monochloropropane—that forms when we heat extracted oil. Many of us cook all vegetables with oil and add oil-based dressings or sauces to almost everything we eat—even the foods that are good for us. All oil contains 120 calories per tablespoon. Oil gets absorbed efficiently and quickly and converted almost instantly into body fat. Even olive oil, coconut oil, and soybean oil. When fat calories are absorbed so rapidly in such a large bolus, they cannot all be utilized for energy, so they are rapidly stored as body fat, something Americans have in large supply. Excess body fat increases the likelihood of cancer. Vegetable oils are calorically dense, low-nutrient foods that contribute to obesity and chronic disease and mess with our immune systems. Similarly, refined grain products like pasta and white bread are poor sources of minerals and vitamins, especially antioxidants. They are also rapidly absorbed and rapidly converted into body fat.

This modern way of eating makes our bodies function at a low efficiency, which stresses our internal organs and in turn leads to chronic disease and premature aging. Though all chronic diseases may have genetic factors contributing to their expression, without the stresses of modern living and modern dietary practices, these weak links in our genetic codes never need to end up as chronic disease.

Chronic diseases have been dramatically on the rise not merely because we're eating an animal-product-based diet, but also because the grains and other plant-derived products we regularly consume are refined and processed, making them nearly devoid of fiber and their essential, but fragile micronutrients. Additionally, we consume an obscene amount of added sweeteners, simple sugars, and, as mentioned, refined vegetable fats or oils. These foods, because they have no significant load of micronutrients and phytochemicals, rob our bodies of our stored micronutrient reserves and add further toxic stress to the body. Consuming empty calories enhances the body's production of free radicals and waste products, which means they cause chronic disease and promote our premature demise.

Most of us consume large quantities of processed foods that are high in fat, salt, sugar, and additives. Instead of a regular diet of fresh fruits, vegetables, beans, nuts, and seeds, which supply the proper nutrients for maximum health, we consume empty calorie after empty calorie. In fact, the top three sources of calories in the SAD today are—shockingly—milk, soda, and margarine, with the combination of fat and refined sugar consisting of 65 percent of our caloric intake.

The USDA's suggested guidelines for almost twenty years—the infamous food pyramid—encouraged a diet that was way too low in plant-based nutrients and fiber. Though USDA recommendations have become significantly better in recent years, they still fail to emphasize fresh fruits, beans, nuts, seeds, and raw and cooked vegetables as the major source of calories. Unrefined plant foods must supply the vast majority of calories for any diet to be safe.

SAD = FAT

Excess body weight has reached epidemic proportions globally, and being overweight is the primary cause of type 2 diabetes; it accelerates atherosclerosis and death from heart disease and has been identified as a strong promoter of cancer. In fact, excess body weight is projected to overtake smoking as the primary cause of cancer in developed countries, as cases of cancer linked to smoking dwindle. Today, two in five

Americans are obese, and the three of five Americans who are not obese are significantly overweight. We are in worse shape today, with heavier bodies and thicker waistlines, than at any time in human history. Refined foods are addicting, and the SAD is making our population too fat.

And yet so-called scientists and nutritionists continue to rally behind erroneous studies, such as a 2013 study—published in the *Journal of the American Medical Association*—that claimed in bold type: "Overweight People Live Longer." But the study was actually a meta-analysis of different studies looking at death in relation to various BMI categories. A person with a BMI between 18.5 and 24.9, for instance, is considered normal, while a person with a BMI between 25 and 29.9 is overweight. A BMI of 30 or more places a person in the obese category. The researchers found a small reduction (6 percent) in the risk of all-cause mortality for overweight people compared with normal people and an 18 percent increase in mortality for obese compared with normal individuals. If a 6-foot male goes from 150 to 220 pounds, his BMI will still be less than 30. This study therefore concluded that a man can gain 70 pounds of fat, and all this weight gain will have no negative effect on his risk of death.

If you believe that, you might as well believe that smoking cigarettes is harmless and eating junk food is fine as long as you take a multivitamin.

This study was essentially worthless because it didn't exclude people with chronic disease recorded at baseline and former smokers. It is well known that illnesses and smoking cause a lower body weight. Sick people always become thinner, while any relatively healthy person who follows the SAD will inevitably become overweight and eventually get sick. If you're eating the SAD and you remain at a normal or near-normal weight, chances are you're either chronically ill or you have an illness yet to be diagnosed.

Current and former smokers, though typically at a lower weight, inevitably die earlier. Any study about body weight and health that doesn't exclude them should automatically be dismissed. Similarly, a number of other medical conditions may also cause unintentional weight loss. These include depression, anxiety, alcoholism, asthma, auto-immune diseases, celiac disease, early pre-diagnosable cancer, chronic obstructive pulmonary disease, depression, drug addiction, and minor to severe digestive disorders, including irritable bowel syndrome.

In this 2013 *JAMA* study, what percentage of the "normal" weight group suffered from one or more of these conditions? The study did not say, but it's likely that many of the study participants were affected by at least one of these conditions. Depression, anxiety, and alcoholism alone could account for the findings in this study, as they affect about 20 percent of the population. But this study was nonetheless triumphantly publicized as "it's okay to be overweight"—exactly what overweight people want to hear.

When people eating the SAD remain at a normal weight, it is often because of disease, not good health. A healthy person eating the SAD should expect to be overweight. Overweight or not, anyone and everyone eating the contemporary SAD is unhealthy, because it is such an unhealthy diet, eventually creating premature, life-threatening disease in all. If you are eating like other Americans and are a normal weight, however, you are most likely battling alcoholism, depression, emotional disorders, undiagnosed cancer, digestive disorders, or auto-immune illness, and your life expectancy may be even more negatively affected.

If this study were correct, then almost every study on fitness, and the benefits of dietary excellence, in the past forty years is wrong! This study is essentially telling us that we should all pack on some extra pounds, exercise less, eat some cheese doodles, and lounge on the couch watching more TV so we can live longer. This is bad science, and because of fatal flaws in the design of the project, it should never have been reported nor published in a major peer-reviewed journal. Especially because other more carefully designed studies, looking at the same issue, show the opposite. The notion that people can be over-weight or obese and still be healthy is a myth. Even the overweight, without high blood pressure, diabetes, or other metabolic abnormalities, still have higher rates of heart attack, stroke, and even cancer if followed long term.

This was confirmed in a recent thorough investigation that pooled together long-term studies compiling the data of more than sixty thousand people that had at least a ten-year follow-up. They found a 24 percent increased risk of heart attack, stroke, and premature death when comparing the "healthy" obese with normal-weight individuals. Even the non-obese overweight had a 21 percent increased chance of premature death compared to normal-weight individuals. The more years the so-called healthy overweight are followed, the more evident it becomes that excess fat on the body is a significant risk for all-cause mortality.[4]

Our waistlines and our weight are the most critical factors governing our health and lifespan. The science behind this fact is indisputable. Despite the overwhelming amount of scientific evidence showing that we could prevent it, people continue to die prematurely after a poor-quality life plagued by sickness and disability. Hardly anyone can escape the lifespan-destructive effects of the SAD, which dramatically increases the risk of developing high blood pressure, diabetes, and heart disease. For instance, the lifetime risk for developing hypertension, or high blood pressure, is more than 90 percent—a 30 percent rise over the past decade. And cardiovascular disease is responsible for approximately 40 percent of all deaths in the United States each year.

There's nothing programmed in our DNA that says we have to get old or fat or develop high blood pressure. We develop high blood pressure because we eat foods high in calories and low in nutrients. And when these calories enter our system without a sufficient amount of protective micronutrients, our cells become congested with free radicals and advanced glycation end products, which can lead to inflammation, cell damage, and premature cell death. High blood pressure, obesity, and heart disease are not natural consequences of aging. They are the result of slow, insidious damage related to years and years of poor dietary choices.

Dietary ignorance, coupled with the addictive nature of refined foods, is now the leading cause of premature death in the modern world. The bottom line is that the majority of Americans ultimately die from their unhealthy nutritional choices. Type 2 diabetes, for instance, a disease born primarily from excess body fat, has exploded, costing our nation a record-high $245 billion in 2012, a 41 percent increase from five years earlier.[5]

Heart disease, diabetes, and most cancers are preventable, but prevention requires change. It sounds simple, and it can be simple once you let knowledge, rather than habits and emotions, guide you. Natural plants, such as vegetables and beans, contain thousands of protective micronutrients, including antioxidants and phytochemicals. When we gain weight, we not only produce more damaging toxic waste in our cells, but we also dilute our body stores of nutrients into a larger pool, lowering the micronutrient concentration in our cells. The simple key to a long, disease-free life is to be relatively thin and well nourished with micronutrients.

The Paleo Diet: Dead Like a Caveman

One of the most popular diets today is also one of the most harmful.

The Paleo crowd believes that if we eat like our Paleolithic ancestors, then we will be much healthier—practically free of disease. All by eating plates and plates of meat.

Well, not only is this the wrong message, it's not even a new message! The high-protein diet continues to take different names and forms, gaining new legions of meat-loving devotees every generation. First it was known as the Atkins diet, then Sugar Busters. Then it came

back as the South Beach diet, and, most recently, the Dukan diet. Now
it's the Paleo diet. Regardless of its name or specific iteration, however,
it's always the same diet—high protein, low carb, enormous risk.

Our modern diet, the SAD, causes diseases. Eating refined sugar,
white flour, processed oils, and commercially processed meats is harmful to our health. But instead of replacing those unhealthy choices with
seeds, nuts, vegetables, fruits, and other foods packed with vital nutrients, the Paleo crowd continues to advocate for more meat. They also
tell you to stay away from beans and whole grains entirely. This is despite irrefutable evidence that eating beans reduces the risk of cancer
and enhances longevity.[6] The Paleo position is diametrically opposed
to the overwhelming scientific evidence that confirms that consuming
large quantities of meat is a health risk.

For a normally sized male, a meat-based Paleo diet contains between
150 and 200 grams of protein a day, or roughly three to four times the
daily amount recommended by the Centers for Disease Control and
Prevention (CDC). This is foolishly and dangerously excessive.

All animal products, including meat, fish, and dairy, are rich in
substances associated with cancer and heart disease: saturated fat,
cholesterol, and arachidonic acid. However, it isn't merely the fat content that makes excessive animal products disease promoting. Animal
protein stimulates the rise of cancer-promoting hormones within the
body, especially insulin-like growth factor-1 (IGF-1). When we consume
animal protein, the body increases its production of IGF-1. Though
IGF-1 is one of the body's most important growth promoters during
infancy and childhood, it accelerates the aging process, promoting the
growth, proliferation, and spread of cancer cells later in life. Elevated
IGF-1 levels are linked to an increased risk of several types of cancers,
including colon, breast, and prostate cancer.[7]

Reduced IGF-1 signaling in adulthood, on the other hand, is associated with reduced oxidative stress, decreased inflammation, enhanced
insulin sensitivity, and longer lifespan.[8]

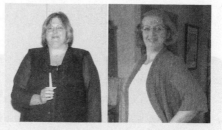

Marcie realized that rapid weight loss is possible and sus-tainable, without deprivation, because, to her pleasant surprise, eating vegetables is far more enjoyable than she ever imagined.

AFTER: Lost 90 pounds in less than a year

It was the beginning of another year and I was (reluctantly) determined to lose weight. I felt terrible and had very little energy. I prayed to God to help me. By the third day of my diet, my husband reconnected with an old employer, who handed him a copy of *Eat to Live*. He said it helped him beat colon cancer. I took this as an answer to my prayers. I read the book and started the nutritarian diet style.

After following the program for about six weeks, I had my lightbulb moment—exactly how Dr. Fuhrman describes it. I began to look forward to eating vegetables. The best part about the nutritarian diet style is that you don't have to weigh your food, and you can actually eat however much you want—all while losing weight! The fact that these foods are found in nature and aren't processed was a huge selling point for me. All of the foods on this diet are what God intended for us to eat.

This plan worked for me when other diets failed, not only because other diets (like Atkins) were hard to maintain, but because depriving and counting calories was just too hard. Of course, the weight coming off rapidly made it easy to continue. Besides the weight loss, I started to think more clearly and focus better. I stopped getting headaches, and I started to enjoy working out. My bouts with depression went away completely. That alone makes it worth staying with this program.

By the fall, I had lost 90 pounds. I can't tell you how wonderful I feel today. Dr. Fuhrman's books are a gift and contain all the research that explains why these foods are so good for us. This knowledge made it easier for me to stick with the plan. Now, I eat for health.

Protein-rich plant foods, such as seeds, beans, and greens, don't raise IGF-1 levels, don't contain pro-inflammatory substances, and are rich in anti-inflammatory and life-extending phytochemicals. The secret to long life and successful weight loss is to get more protein from natural plant sources and less from animal products.

Clearly, at this point in nutritional science we have enough studies which show that diets higher in the amount of meat shorten lifespan and promote cancer. And these studies have been consistent in various regions of the world and with various types of meat, implicating many different aspects of meat, including grass-fed meats and the more contaminated commercial corn-fed or grain-fed meats.

But you'd never hear this if you're talking to a Paleo diet advocate. Recently, I attended a medical conference in Denver, Colorado, where I heard Loren Cordain, an exercise physiologist and leader of the Paleo movement, give a talk. In his presentation, he advocated a diet in which 80 percent of calories come from meat. I couldn't believe what I was hearing. That is more than double the high meat intake that Americans already consume! How could he advocate such a cancer-promoting diet? When an astute conference attendee asked Cordain about IGF-1, he replied, irritably and incorrectly, "Only sugar raises IGF-1 levels, not meat." Never mind science; Cordain was staying on message, though he didn't deny the cancer-promoting effects of elevating IGF-1. That animal protein is the primary driver of higher IGF-1 levels is a fly in the ointment that all Paleo advocates must acknowledge. The clarity of the scientific studies on this issue shows that their favored diet promotes cancer.

A recent scientific study compared the amount of animal products consumed in 157 different countries with high-quality food consumption and disease-occurrence data and noted that cancer rates were highest (with a fifteen- to twenty-five-year lag time) in populations consuming the most animal products and lowest in those consuming the least. Fewer than 10 percent of calories from animal products correlated with lowest cancer risks (standardized for age).[9]

Though some people may experience moderate, short-term weight loss by reducing refined carbohydrates and increasing calories from animal products, such as poultry and other meats, the dramatically dangerous health results are clear over the long term. A number of recent studies confirm this. The Nurses' Health Study and Health Professionals Follow-up Study, for instance, found a positive association between a diet high in animal protein and cardiovascular mortality.[10] A diet consisting mostly of vegetable sources of protein shared no such link with cardiovascular mortality. Similarly, the Health Professionals Follow-up Study also showed a causal relationship between strokes and ischemic, or coronary, heart disease and a high-protein, low-carb diet.[11]

A huge Swedish prospective study also gathered data from more than forty thousand women between the ages of thirty and forty-nine.[12] Researchers followed them for an average of 15.7 years. Women with a diet low in carbohydrates and high in animal protein significantly increased their risk of cardiovascular disease, ischemic heart disease, and ischemic stroke in a dose-dependent manner (that is, these diseases rose in proportion to the increased consumption of animal protein).

Researchers also found that for every increase of 5 grams of animal protein and decrease of 20 grams of carbohydrates a day, the risk of cardiovascular disease was increased by 5 percent. The increased consumption of meat has consistently been associated with an increased incidence in type 2 diabetes as well. Even half a serving more of meat a day increased the risk of diabetes by 48 percent in a large study of almost 150,000 individuals.[13]

The EPIC-PANACEA study, one of the largest weight evaluation studies in history, found that meat and poultry intake, after adjustment for calories, was responsible for the highest amount of body fat.[14] What this means is a person who eats meat will weigh more and have more body fat than someone whose source of calories is predominantly from plants, even though the number of calories is *exactly* the same.

The data are overwhelming. Clearly, we need to eat much less animal products.

The only real controversial or unclear issue here is what amount of animal products is safe and which types are best. Many people believe that seafood is the most favorable animal product to consume, but given the high concentration of pollutants in most seafood, this is not so clear. Wild-caught animal products are definitely cleaner sources and are therefore preferred. Still, less is almost always more. The less animal products we consume, the lower the risk of disease. This is seen even when we consider the cleanest, most natural animal products, because the concentration of animal protein is the main feature that promotes abnormal cell growth and disease.

The Adventist Health Study had the best-controlled data for shedding some light on this subject. It compared vegans with flexitarians, that is, people who eat meat only a few times a week. It showed the vegans had an average increased lifespan of 1.5 years compared to the flexitarians eating one or two servings of animal products a week, which is less than 5 percent of total calories.[15] Recently, I have been advocating either a vegan diet or a diet with less than 5 percent of calories from animal products. I think the evidence is now compelling enough to show that even 10 percent, which I had suggested as the upper limit in the past, may be too much animal products to optimally protect against cancer, largely because it could add roughly 200 calories from animal products and more than 30 grams of animal protein to your diet a day. Such a level could elevate IGF-1 levels beyond what is optimal in most people.

Regardless of this debatable point of interest, and the difficulty in establishing a precise percentage of safety, it is irresponsible and negligent to advise people to increase their consumption of animal products from 30 percent up to 60 to 80 percent, as Paleo and other high-protein advocates do. No reasonable scientist familiar with the body of literature on this subject would consider this amount safe. I think nutritional scientists the world over would agree that we have to reduce the level of 30 percent by at least half, not increase it.

Even the dangerous Paleo diet may look acceptable when compared with the SAD. However, only a diet style rich in colorful vegetables, both raw and cooked, can ward off disease, reduce fat storage, protect against cardiovascular disease and cancer, and simultaneously stabilize your weight. The Paleo diet is a passing fad that caters to the like-minded meat-obsessed crowd, helping them justify how they want to eat. Every new iteration of high-protein mania succeeds despite the cumulative evidence of thousands of studies that consistently shows that the relative healthfulness of any diet is generally proportional to its higher vegetable content and the variety of its vegetable content. Paleo and high-protein diets are only for people who still believe the earth is flat.

It is also worth noting that some Paleo advocates will tell the story that they experienced a "failure to thrive" on a vegan or vegetarian diet. They may report that their body was falling apart and they were dying until they started eating more animal products again. Of course, they didn't try eating higher-protein plant food and more whole-plant fats from high-protein seeds and nuts or even some limited amount of animal products in conjunction with more beans. To feel well, they just had to go back to eating lots and lots of meat. These stories merely indicate bias and nutritional ignorance of how to structure a healthy diet and how to achieve nutritional adequacy for a wide range of human needs and requirements. Even those people who require a diet with more protein and fat can achieve that without resorting to a diet loaded with meat. As you can see in Tables 1 and 2 on the following page, beans, seeds, nuts, and greens are all high in protein.

TABLE 1. SAMPLE PLANT PROTEIN CONTENT (GRAMS)

28.6	Soybeans, boiled (1 cup)
24.0	Mediterranean pine nuts (½ cup)
18.2	Almonds (3 oz.)
17.9	Lentils, boiled (1 cup)
15.3	Kidney beans, boiled (1 cup)
15.2	Spinach, frozen (2 cups)
14.5	Chickpeas, boiled (1 cup)
13.2	Hemp seeds (½ cup)
12.8	Sesame seeds (½ cup)
11.5	Sunflower seeds (½ cup)
11.4	Broccoli, frozen (2 cups)
11.0	Tofu, extra firm (4 oz.)
10.3	Collards, boiled (2 cups)
8.2	Peas, frozen (1 cup)

TABLE 2. SAMPLE ANIMAL PROTEIN CONTENT (GRAMS)

26.2	Chicken (light meat, roasted, 3 oz.)
21.6	Salmon (Atlantic, wild, broiled, 3 oz.)
19.8	Beef short loin (Porterhouse, ⅛-in. fat, broiled, 3 oz.)
12.6	Eggs (2)
8.2	Milk, 1% (1 cup)

My broad experience as a physician has demonstrated that occasionally a vegan diet may need tweaking for people who have higher fat and protein needs. But these individuals are rare, and such additional requirements can most often be met while maintaining a vegan diet. In the rare instances that it can't, however, a small amount of animal products should suffice.

The amino acid that repeatedly comes up borderline or low when I test levels on vegans who are not quite feeling up to snuff is taurine.

Additional taurine is often helpful for these individuals. The only other nutrients low or borderline low with a diet without animal products are B_{12}, zinc, iodine, and the marine fats eicosapentaenoic acid (EPA) and docosahexaenoic acid (DHA), all of which are easily supplemented. Of course, vitamin D, the "sunshine vitamin," also has to be considered because deficiencies are common and can lead to serious health problems.

I am lobbying for broad acceptance of basic nutritional principles by everyone, so people can all respect the healthiest dietary style. The only question is the level of compliance. There shouldn't be a dramatic chasm between one dietary camp and another because nutritional science isn't that controversial anymore. A nutritarian diet, as described in this book, is high in whole plant food. It pays close attention to broad nutritional diversity and allows for limited animal products, as desired by an individual. Competing dieting principles should come to an end, because there are no legitimate arguments against the preponderance of evidence that exists today.

The Mediterranean Mistake: Olive Oil and Pasta Are Not Health Foods

The Mediterranean diet describes a cuisine with certain characteristics common to countries bordering the Mediterranean Sea. Traditionally, these cuisines are heavy in plants and include lots of fruits, vegetables, cereals, legumes, and nuts. Red meat is rarely consumed, and chicken and fish appear only in small amounts. Yogurt and cheese are used as condiments, and red wine is consumed regularly.

The climate and soil surrounding the Mediterranean Sea produce a wide spectrum of high-nutrient plants, including broccoli, tomatoes, grapes, figs, walnuts, and olives. The beneficial effects of the Mediterranean diet are due to antioxidant-rich foods, including vegetables, fruits, and beans as well as lots of onions and garlic. The increased amount of broccoli, nuts, and beans, for instance, coupled with the heavy use of tomatoes in most meals, make most Mediterranean dishes rich in phyto-chemicals, which accounts for its protective effects. And the use of fish instead of meat helps decrease the consumption of saturated fat, while helping to increase the level of beneficial omega-3 fatty acids. Nuts, es-pecially walnuts, are also commonly used in dishes. Beneficial health effects have been noted from the use of even small amounts of walnuts in the diet. Numerous studies have shown that people who eat walnuts regularly have half the heart disease rates of those who rarely eat them.[16]

For these reasons, as well as the powerful health benefits of tomato sauce and other tomato products, it is easy to understand why the Mediterranean diet is widely considered healthful compared to the SAD. Beneficial health outcomes are also evident in other areas of the world, such as Japan, rural China, Fiji, and Tibet. People in these regions have substantially lower rates of heart disease, cancer, and obesity, and their elderly people are healthier and live longer, compared to in the United States. We can learn about the positive aspects of all these culturally di-verse diets and utilize their culinary principles to make a diet deliciously varied and even more disease-protective than the Mediterranean diet. However, we do not want to replicate the drawbacks and unhealthful aspects of these regional cuisines, such as white rice in the Chinese diet, white pasta in the Mediterranean diet, and high salt intake in the Japanese diet.

The reality is that modern fast-food outlets and processed food industries have permeated most of the modern world. Mediterranean people now follow a diet much like our own, and the rates of heart dis-ease and obesity are skyrocketing in these countries. In Italy, the diet they follow today does not follow the guidelines of the old-time, health-ful Mediterranean style. They eat much like we do, eating more cheese and fewer vegetables than before. They now have the same high preva-lence of high cholesterol levels and heart attack risk as Americans.[17]

Certainly the white flour pasta in the Mediterranean diet is not something we want to include in our own. It is just as bad for you as white bread. In fact, there is almost no chemical difference between the two. Both are made with white refined flour, which has been linked to diabetes, obesity, heart disease, and various cancers. White flour actually makes your blood sugar levels rise almost as much as plain sugar. Carbohydrates—literally chains of sugar molecules—are found in all plants and foods made from plants. They can be a single sugar or three of four bound together, but when thousands of sugars are bound together, they are called *starch*. When these simple carbon molecules are bound together so tightly that your body can't break them down and digest them, they are called *fiber*.

When your digestive enzymes break down the carbohydrates into simple glucose molecules, they enter the body just as if you had sucked on a sugar cube. All the white starches—white bread, white rice, white pasta, and even white potatoes—are rapidly converted to glucose, or sugar, which is absorbed into the bloodstream almost instantaneously. When blood sugar levels go skyrocketing, it overworks the pancreas as it tries to match the load of sugar with a large amount of insulin. Not only is this stressful to the body and the pancreas, but metabolizing that large energy load without a concomitant intake of micronutrients creates metabolic havoc in the cells. Toxic metabolites build up in cells when we consume calories without antioxidant and phytochemical micronutrients needed to remove and control the toxic by-products of metabolism. So as we eat more low-nutrient and low-fiber carbohydrates, we build up more cell toxicity, leading to disease and food addiction.

Indeed, eating sugar and white flour not only leads to diabetes, but both of these foodstuffs are also linked to cancer. Quite a few studies have linked the consumption of high-glycemic, low-nutrient food to cancer. One such study showed more than a 200 percent increase in the risk of breast cancer in women whose diets are more than half refined carbohydrates.[18]

Oil: From your lips to your hips.

Whereas most of the fat in the SAD comes from cheese, butter, and meat—all of which contain dangerous *trans* fats—the principal source of fat in the Mediterranean diet is olive oil, a monounsaturated fat. Foods rich in monounsaturated fats are less harmful than foods full of saturated fats and *trans* fats, but that doesn't mean they're "healthful."

Like sugar, oil is a processed food, which means that its nutrients and fiber have been removed. Walnut oil, for instance, has a vastly different biological effect than raw walnuts, and sesame seed oil has a different biological effect than sesame seeds. Whole nuts and seeds release their calories over hours, not minutes, and have unique health benefits. All oil, including olive oil, contains 120 calories per tablespoon of rapidly absorbed fat. Those tablespoons of fat calories can add up fast. In fact, the average American consumes about 400 calories of oil a day—a large contributor to high body fat. Many people use the favorable reputation of the Mediterranean diet as an excuse to pour more olive oil on their food. Ounce for ounce, oil is one of the most fattening, calorically dense foods on the planet. It packs more calories per pound (4,020) than butter (3,200). Simply put, a lot of oil means a lot of empty calories. And an excess of empty calories means an excess of weight, which can lead to diabetes, high blood pressure, stroke, heart disease, and many forms of cancer.

Certainly, it's better to use olive oil than butter or margarine, but this feature of the Mediterranean diet easily can sabotage your weight-loss results. Using oil in the preparation of meals will make losing weight more difficult, and many people won't lose weight at all. A small amount of olive oil would be acceptable in an otherwise high-nutrient diet if a person were thin and physically active. For many overweight individuals, however, oil adds another 300 to 700 calories to their daily menu. Those low-nutrient calories impede the goal of superior health and weight loss, especially when seeds and nuts are the preferable source of fat calories. To continue to eat foods prepared in oil and maintain a healthful, slender figure, dieters must carefully count calories and eat tiny portions—not something I recommend because it cycles dieters back to a cycle of failure, as they try to consume only thimble-size portions of food.

In addition to taking up most of a dieter's caloric intake, oil significantly lowers his or her intake of nutrients and fiber. Compared with its high caloric content, olive oil contains very few nutrients, other than a small amount of vitamin E and a negligible amount of phytochemical compounds. It's true that in the past, Mediterranean people regularly ate olive oil, but they also worked hard in the fields, walking about nine miles a day, often while guiding a heavy plow.

When reading about the Mediterranean diet, most Americans don't take home the message to eat loads of tomato sauce, vegetables, beans, and fruits and to exercise. They blindly accept the myth that olive oil is a health food. Then they coat everything with cheese, one of the most fattening foods on the planet, and think they are eating healthfully.

The villain isn't fat in general, but rather oils, saturated fats, *trans* fats, and the fats consumed in processed foods. A healthful alternative to olive oil are nuts and seeds, which contain fewer calories per tablespoon than oil. At the same time, the body doesn't absorb all of the fat calories of nuts and seeds. Plus, the fats in nuts and seeds are slowly absorbed, satiating hunger. They stabilize blood glucose at a low level, reducing fat-storage hormones and encouraging your body to burn fat for its energy needs. Nuts and seeds are also rich in antioxidants and phytochemicals, and when eaten with other nutrient-rich foods, they increase the absorption of phytochemicals and antioxidants from those foods as well. They offer unique health benefits that effectively protect against heart disease and cancer.[19]

Nuts and seeds are also a plant-food source of protein. Nuts and seeds (and avocados) are natural plant sources of the healthful fats we need. Fats in nuts and seeds are rich in sterols, stanols, fibers, minerals, lignans, and other health-promoting nutrients that help lower cholesterol. They are linked in numerous scientific studies to a slimmer waistline and longer lifespan.

Researchers have found that including nuts and seeds in your diet can help you lose weight. Although they aren't low in calories and are relatively high in fat, eating them may actually satisfy hunger and suppress appetite. I find that eating a small amount of nuts or seeds helps dieters feel satiated, stay with the program, and have more success at long-term weight loss. Seeds give you all the advantages of nuts, plus more. They are generally higher in protein than nuts and have many additional, important nutrients, such as omega-3 fatty acids and anti-cancer lignans (which will be discussed later).

A recent study compared a traditional Mediterranean diet with one that substituted nuts for oil. According to the study, the Mediterranean diet minus the nuts did not lessen atherosclerotic plaque. The version that substituted nuts for the oil, however, did.[20] The Mediterranean diet was further evaluated in Spain, randomizing 7,216 men and women to include either nuts or olive oil. The group consuming more than three servings of nuts per week had a 39 percent reduced all-cause mortality over the average 4.8 years of follow-up, compared with the group not consuming nuts.[21]

Today, people who live along the Mediterranean are overweight, just like us. They still eat lots of olive oil, but their consumption of fruits, vegetables, and beans is down. Meat, cheese, and fish consumption has risen, while their level of physical activity has plummeted. They have become more like Americans. Utilize the healthful aspects of the Mediterranean diet, but leave behind its weaknesses so that you don't merely reduce heart disease and obesity a little bit, but eliminate them altogether. Even people with a family history of heart disease can be free of heart disease forever with a nutritarian diet.

Wheat: How Worried
Should We Really Be?

In his popular book *Wheat Belly,* William Davis, M.D., advises people to avoid wheat products entirely. He contends that modern "genetically altered" wheat is the main reason our society is sick and overweight. By genetically altered, he doesn't mean genetically modified; instead, he merely refers to the cross-breeding of wheat cells over the years. This, according to Davis, is the chief cause of diabetes, heart disease, and the nation's obesity epidemic. He lets off the hook sugar, white rice, soda, oil, fried potatoes, bacon, commercial meats, and cheeseburgers, placing the blame predominantly on wheat.

Throughout the book, Davis attributes negative qualities to "wheat" but then proceeds to demonstrate and reference the negative effects of white flour, a highly processed form of whole wheat. His lack of precision here is confusing and not scientific. The more finely you grind a grain into flour, the higher its glycemic load becomes. Whole wheat pastry flour, for instance, has a higher glycemic index than coarsely ground whole grains, which are more glycemic than intact whole grains such as boiled wheat kernels, sprouted wheat, or wheat berries. Davis is not making it clear if wheat is the issue, or the way we process and manufacture flour.

The claim that wheat is the villain is misleading because most of the data Davis presents to vilify wheat demonstrates that it's actually white flour that's the problem—not all wheat. For example, he presented data from the China-Cornell-Oxford Project to show a correlation between increasing consumption of wheat flour and modern disease, but he failed to mention that people in the study were eating products made from white flour, not whole grains.

Contrary to Davis's claims, wheat hasn't morphed into a toxic monster food. It is simply too often overly processed and overly ground,

which jacks up its glycemic levels. It then quickly empties out its calories into the body, spiking our insulin levels. Bagels, pancakes, muffins, bread, rolls, cake, pretzels, pizza, breakfast cereals, and pasta are
all made from white flour, which is absorbed into the bloodstream as
quickly as sugar. White flour and other processed grains promote diabetes, obesity, heart disease, and cancer. Add these to all the soda, sweets,
oils, cheeses, meats, and other processed junk food that Americans
consume, and it's no wonder our population is sick and overweight.

However, Davis contends that even a little whole wheat product
in the diet is too immune-system stimulating and can keep you from
weight loss and optimal health. Is that the case? Is wheat more glycemic
than all the other grains? Is even a moderate amount of real whole
grain wheat really so bad for the majority of people who have no problem with gluten? That is clearly a fairy tale. As long as whole grains are
in the same form, their glycemic effect is very similar. Davis implicates
wheat as the villain because it contains more of the starch amylopectin A, which is more glycemic than amylopectin B and C. But the study
he references for this data actually shows that all the other measured
whole grains—oats, brown rice, and barley—share similar amounts of
rapidly digestible amylopectin A.

Davis also states that wheat is more glycemic than pure sugar.
This is more nonsense. In fact, the glycemic load of sucrose (200
calories) is 37.2, while the glycemic load of whole wheat bread (200
calories, three slices) is 26.1. What's more, whole wheat kernels, the
preferred way to consume wheat, have a relatively low glycemic load
of 13.5.

Davis makes a number of other unsubstantiated claims to boost
his contention that wheat is dangerous. While pointing out the very
real health hazards of wheat to people with gluten intolerance and
celiac disease, he fails to qualify his statement against the extremely
low number of people in these two categories. The prevalence of
wheat allergies in the United States, for instance, is found in only 0.4

percent of the population, while celiac disease is found in less than 1 percent of the population.[22] Nonceliac gluten sensitivity doesn't yet have a distinct definition, but the current estimate is 6 percent of Americans.[23] Without quantifying the number of people who have these difficulties, Davis ends up only inciting in the wider public an irrational and unsubstantiated fear of wheat. Certainly, people with celiac disease or gluten intolerance can experience severe health problems if they eat wheat, but that is ancillary to the core message of his book—mainly, that wheat makes us fat and is dangerous to our health, even though Davis doesn't present the science to back up such claims.

To make matters worse, he compounds his errors by advocating a diet of unlimited helpings of meat, oil, eggs, and fish, just as his partners in the Paleo and other high-animal-protein diets do. He even goes so far as to claim that animal products and saturated fat are only tangentially associated with heart disease, telling his readers that they can eat all the high-saturated-fat meats and cheeses they want as long as they cut out wheat entirely from their diet. I was flabbergasted. While Davis also urges his readers to make "vegetables, in all their wondrous variety," a centerpiece of their diets, he fails to make room for "the best foods on the planet earth" (as we agree vegetables are) next to the unlimited helpings of meat, eggs, cheese, and oils. I guess he doesn't see that readers will have to reduce the intake of some other less desirable foods significantly in order to eat lots of vegetables, beans, nuts, seeds, and fruit.

Davis takes the extreme position that wheat and processed foods are the singular villains, ignoring how the deadly combination of processed wheat, processed foods, *and* too much animal products are scientifically shown to lead to weight gain, diabetes, heart disease, cancer, premature aging, and dementia. Like everyone else behind almost every fad diet, Davis has to exaggerate and misrepresent the data on hand to make them fit his biases.

Low-Fat Fallacies

Antiscientific thinking also permeates the vegan community, perpetu-ated by some well-known vegan health authors and respected authori-ties within its ranks. Unfortunately, most authorities have their own predetermined biases. People interested in true science-based nutrition have no predetermined dietary agenda and are open to modifying future recommendations for improvement; they inquisitively seek out and admit problems that may develop, changing recommendations accordingly. All too often, vegans in positions of authority look for and report only scientific support for veganism, ignoring evidence or clini-cal experience that contradicts their teachings. Similar to the resistant high-protein crowd, vegan leaders too often hang their reputations on past pronouncements and are therefore reticent to change them as better science and more conclusive evidence becomes available. This resistance perpetuates disagreements within the health science com-munity and slows education about and acceptance of healthful eating.

It also leaves some individuals who are following their recommen-dations unsatisfied and not adequately cared for. These people do not thrive when trying to avoid all fats in an attempt to maintain a fat per-cent of below 10 percent in their diet. Some individuals have unique digestive and absorptive requirements that call for slight modifications in their dietary standards. Most commonly, a small percentage of in-dividuals have higher fat needs or higher protein needs, as do many rapidly growing children, serious athletes, and pregnant and nursing women. Importantly, genetic differences in fatty acid metabolism also need to be recognized.

About thirty years ago, for instance, some vegan health enthusi-asts hypothesized that the benefits of a vegan diet stemmed from the fact that this diet was so low in fat. An extremely low-fat vegan diet quickly began to receive significant media exposure as it was clinically demonstrated to prevent and reverse heart disease. Fat, then, became the dietary *villain du jour*. The more fat you could avoid, the leaders of this community argued, the better. This viewpoint seemed reasonable at the time, largely because the scientific studies on fat consumption back then (showing negative health effects) always investigated the effects of consuming processed oils and animal fats. (They had yet to investigate the results of populations consuming more fat from whole seeds and nuts.) It therefore wasn't unreasonable to assume that the main benefit of a vegan diet came from the avoidance of fat in general. Many vegans embraced a low-fat vegan diet, eschewing all oils and almost all seeds and nuts, trying to keep their fat intake below 10 percent of calories.

A report in 1990 seemed to confirm the value of this way of eating. Dean Ornish, a physician and founder of the Preventive Medicine Research Institute in Sausalito, California, published the Lifestyle Heart Trial, which showed that 82 percent of the experimental group following a very low-fat, mostly vegan diet had demonstrated regression of their obstructive coronary atherosclerotic lesions.[24] This means that for the majority of subjects, this diet style reversed heart disease. This landmark study forced people to accept the reality that heart disease can be reversed with aggressive nutritional intervention. Ornish and his colleagues showed that comprehensive lifestyle changes can help reduce even severe coronary atherosclerosis after only one year, all without the use of lipid-lowering drugs. Soon, others around the country, such as Caldwell B. Esselstyn, M.D., started using similar extremely low-fat vegan diets with impressive results.[25]

Even though these physicians advocating extremely low-fat vegan diets have helped thousands of people and revolutionized the treatment of heart disease, some questions remain. Is it helpful to scare people with heart disease away from eating a few walnuts? Does this advice to avoid unsalted nuts and seeds offer any added benefit to the vegan diet style? And, can excluding all nuts and seeds even be harmful for some people? Accumulating evidence from scientific clinical trials, epidemiological studies, and my clinical findings led me to take a slightly different approach.

Following these well-publicized protocols, I was called on to care for many in this newfound community of low-fat vegan dieters with advanced heart disease. Hundreds of them came to me for additional guidance because they had complaints and questions. Some of them exhibited symptoms of fatty acid deficiency such as depression, dry skin, fatigue, poor recovery after exercise, and cardiac arrhythmias like premature ventricular contractions. I even examined patients who developed atrial fibrillation after adopting this extremely low-fat vegan approach to eating.

A certain amount of essential fatty acids is required for hormonal production and healthy cell membranes. They are also necessary to maintain cell integrity, permeability, shape, and flexibility; and they are critical for the development and functioning of the heart, brain, and nervous system. A deficiency in fat can compromise the absorption of fat-soluble vitamins and minerals, such as carotenoids, vitamin E, zinc, and manganese as well as the anticancer phytochemicals found in vegetables. This deficiency can also exacerbate the general poor absorption of zinc that can result from a vegan diet because whole grains, nuts, and legumes bind to zinc, inhibiting its absorption.

By incorporating nuts and seeds back into my vegan patients' diets, as well as by supplementing these diets with low doses of DHA—a long-chain omega-3 fatty acid usually found in fish but also available as an algae-derived vegan supplement—I was able to generally cure their symptoms and bring up the low levels of these fatty acids shown in their blood tests.

Thousands of my patients, clients, and readers reclaimed their favorable weights and reversed their atherosclerosis. Many are now thriving in their eighties and nineties, with no signs of slowing down. Their cholesterol is low. They aren't hypertensive. Their hearts are in great condition, and they're all off medications for heart disease.

My protocol worked, but unfortunately, some people who adopted the extremely low-fat vegan diet felt so poorly they eventually went back to eating excessive amounts of animal products again. These experiences were reported to me by some of these individuals, and one can find such complaints across the Internet and in articles and books. Fortunately, I had the opportunity to work with many of these people and turn them around to healthful eating with a diet that worked well for them. With a slight tweak of their diets, they were able to remain vegan.

Over the past thirty years, evidence on the benefits of consuming nuts and seeds has accumulated. It is now too definitive to ignore. Scores of studies have demonstrated that nuts and seeds help decrease dramatically the occurrence of cancer, heart disease, and strokes, while significantly increasing the average person's life expectancy.

I recently made a list of seventy-seven new studies on nuts and seeds. They all show positive effects on weight, health, and longevity. While these studies are far too intensive to discuss in full here, I will highlight some interesting points. As people ate more fat calories from seeds and nuts, instead of cooked carbohydrates such as potatoes, rice, and bread, their blood glucose levels dropped. So did their weight. In other words, people who ate more nuts and seeds demonstrated a lower weight and thinner waist than those eating fewer calories.[26] Certainly, one shouldn't eat too many nuts because they are rich in calories. In reasonable quantities, however, they increase stool fat (the amount of fat the body doesn't absorb) and help control overeating.

In fact, the Harvard Nurses' Health Study, which involved more than ten thousand women, now followed for more than thirty-five years, found that nuts and seeds shared the strongest link to longevity. Eating two small handfuls a week, according to the study, had as many lifespan-enhancing benefits as jogging four hours a week.[27]

This evidence was also clear in a study of Seventh-Day Adventists published in 2001.[28] The study, which followed thirty-four thousand vegans and near-vegans for twelve years, found that the people who lived the longest regularly consumed nuts and seeds. Those who didn't had a higher rate of all-cause mortality. Even those whose diet included a small amount of animal products and also used seeds and nuts outlived vegans who did not eat seeds and nuts.

And yet there are still two extremes. On one side are people who believe that eating an excess of animal products and animal fat is the only way to survive. On the other are people who resist eating *any* type of fat. It seems you can be only for or against fat—a startling polarity that cheats both camps from getting the most nutritional benefit from eating healthier. Both extremes may also result in potential health difficulties later in life.

Take, for instance, the thorny issue of EPA and DHA supplementation within the low-fat vegan community. EPA and DHA, two long-chain fatty acids, are essential to fetal development, cardiovascular function, and the prevention of dementia. The only problem is that the richest source of EPA and DHA is fatty fish. While it's perfectly reasonable—and perfectly healthy—to avoid fatty fish for a number of reasons, there are still a number of health benefits to including omega-3 fatty acids in our regular diet. Most advocates of a low-fat vegan diet refute this view and resist findings that may contradict their opinions, as if their minds are already closed. It almost seems that they are resistant to recognizing that many people may need a source of DHA fat, because that would mean that a vegan diet is not the best natural diet for man. For some in this community, it looks like their philosophical preferences cloud their judgment of the available evidence. When there are only a limited number of long-term trials available, we have to rely more on clinical evidence and be cautious so all people's individual health needs are considered.

While EPA acts to increase cerebral blood flow via eicosanoids (messengers in the nervous system), DHA increases membrane fluidity, which enables membrane function and signaling properties. DHA also increases the growth of neurons and the uptake of glucose in the brain, important steps in neurotransmission, and helps promote neuronal survival while protecting the brain from degeneration.

Cognitive decline in the elderly is often marked by a decrease in plasma DHA levels. A report from the Framingham Heart Study, for instance, showed that people with plasma DHA levels in the top quartile of values had a significantly lower risk (47 percent) of developing all-cause dementia than those in the bottom quartile.[29] Other studies have corroborated this, demonstrating a linear relationship between the intake of DHA and EPA and the prevention of cognitive decline.[30]

Similarly, patients suffering from Alzheimer's disease show a lower content of DHA in the gray matter of the frontal lobe and hippocampus of the brain than patients who don't have Alzheimer's.[31] Epidemiological and animal studies also suggest that omega-3 fatty acids protect against cognitive decline.[32]

At the same time, a two-year study demonstrated that DHA and EPA supplementation improved memory.[33] These findings were corroborated in another randomized placebo-controlled trial with subjects who had habitually low intakes of fish and seafood.[34] Over a six-month period, the participants consumed either 1 gram of DHA per day or a placebo. Their cognitive performance was tested before and after the intervention. Those taking DHA supplements improved their memory and cognitive reaction times.

More recently, DHA has been linked to depression. Vegans with strikingly low levels of omega-3 EPA and DHA, for instance, are more at risk for depression, postpartum depression, and/or neurological decline later in life. A large study of eight hundred suicides, for example, found that the likelihood of suicide was 62 percent higher in people with low levels of DHA. What's more, a 14 percent increase in the risk of suicide death came with each standard deviation below normal DHA levels.[35] Interventional studies of people with major depression have shown omega-3 fatty acids to be effective in fighting depression.[36]

Having served as the primary physician since the early 1970s for this community of vegans eating a healthy, whole food–based diet, as well as raw food vegans since the early 1990s, I am in a unique position to point out how such a rigid ideology can sometimes prevent someone from reaching optimal health. Some people even refused to take vitamin B_{12}, a separate but serious issue, resulting in the death of some staunch philosophical naturalists. However, this experience enabled me to observe and investigate the cause of neurological problems that developed in this community that were not secondary to B_{12} deficiency, by checking their level of omega-3 fatty acids.

A pattern emerged in those with later-life neurological decline: when I then checked their DHA levels, they were either extremely low or undetectable. I have since tested blood levels of scores of vegans and found similar deficiencies in many, even if they were consuming adequate amounts of alpha-linolenic acid (ALA), the short-chain omega-3 fatty acid found in appreciable quantity in walnuts, hemp and chia seeds, flaxseeds, and soybeans.

On its own, ALA is an inefficient source of DHA because its effect depends on its conversion first to EPA and then to DHA. This conversion varies considerably from person to person. Vegans who consume adequate sources of ALA still regularly exhibit low levels of EPA and, in particular, DHA. A trial of 165 nonsupplemented healthy vegans demonstrated this clearly.[37] Their mean red blood cell omega-3 index was 3.7, which indicated that the majority of the group suffered from suboptimal levels.

More concerning was that 27 percent showed levels below 3, a more serious deficiency, and 8.5 percent of participants showed an index below 2.5, a severe and potentially dangerous deficiency. Some people point to the dangers of high-dose supplementation with fish oil or of eating too much fish as reasons to not recommend any such supplements. It's important to always remember that as with any nutrient, both too little and too much can be harmful. Recognizing the potential risk of excess and avoiding excess is not a justification for remaining deficient.

Even though the existing science is not yet 100 percent definitive on the clinical implications of these deficiencies, enough evidence exists to show that EPA and DHA are semi-essential nutrients. I believe that people who abstain from eating fish, for whatever reason—personal, health, or ideological—should supplement their diets with low doses of EPA and DHA, or at least have a blood test to make sure that no significant deficiency exists. Ignoring this could place a person at significant risk later in life. Which is why I recommend that, if you cannot assure adequacy with blood work, non-fish eaters, vegans, and flexitarians take a low-dose algae supplement of about 200 milligrams of EPA and DHA per day, with at least 100 milligrams from the DHA component, to help prevent cognitive decline. As an alternative, I recommend one purified fish oil supplement every other day. A low-dose supplement can prevent deficiency and effectively raise red blood cell membrane fatty acid balance as measured with blood tests.[38]

Some thought leaders in the vegan community disagree with and adamantly discourage following even this conservative recommendation, ignoring the nutritional and dietary needs of individuals who don't fit into their one-size-fits-all rigid dietary paradigm. But there is simply no good reason to blindly adhere to an extremely low-fat vegan diet. No human population in the history of the earth has lived on an extremely low-fat vegan diet or any diet so radically low in fat. Science has shown that such a diet is far from ideal and can sometimes lead to disease. At the very least, it might prevent achieving optimal health and longevity, the ultimate goal of any diet style.

Yet many in this community are passionately attached to the "wisdom" of their preferred superstar doctors or to their desire to support animal rights or other altruistic advantages of a vegan diet. They have embraced leaders in the movement because of the reputations of those leaders and their support of veganism, but the fact remains: nuts and seeds are important for protection against cancer and a heart disease–related death.[39] Inevitably, this extreme anti-fat dietary position will fade out of favor with time, as most incorrect dietary patterns usually do. More and more nutritional scientists are recognizing that fat isn't always the villain it was once made out to be.

Just Eat

The bottom line is that you needn't adopt any extreme fad diet; instead, eat lots of natural plant foods. Forget fat. Forget carbohydrates. Don't worry about carbohydrate-to-protein ratios and—for your own sake—please ditch the diets. We need to stop the low-fat extremism, high-protein extremism, low-carb extremism, high-carb extremism, and high-fat extremism (believe it or not, this is gaining popularity too). None of this is constructive to solving our nation's confusion and dietary quagmire.

Good nutrition meets, without excess, your macronutrient needs (fat, carbohydrate, and protein—the three sources of calories) and provides for sufficient micronutrients (vitamins, minerals, and phytochemicals—the parts of food that don't contain calories). A broad range of macronutrients in your diet is acceptable, provided that you're not overloading on calories—particularly empty calories that keep you locked in the vicious cycle of food addiction, toxic hunger, and overeating.

Health is the first consideration; weight is secondary. Focusing on health and a better quality of life is the only consistent way to maintain a favorable weight. To achieve an optimal amount of phytonutrients and other micronutrients, all you have to do is eat a large amount of vegetables every day. When you eat lots of vegetables, especially green vegetables, you meet your body's need for fiber and micronutrients without having to consume too many calories. To balance out your diet and fill your daily caloric needs, choose an assortment of other foods that have protective health benefits—foods such as tomatoes, berries, beans, seeds, and mushrooms. Eat more fruits, beans, squash, peas, lentils, soybeans, nuts, and seeds. And less bread, potato, and rice—especially white rice.

Stop looking for diets and just eat as healthfully as possible. You know what healthful eating means, and if you eat healthfully enough, you won't need to diet. No matter how popular they are, diets simply don't work. So don't diet. Eat only for health. It is important to thoroughly understand how harmful diets are for you and your health, which is the subject of the next chapter.

CHAPTER THREE

The End of Dieting

If we all understood that the secret to superior health and a long life was a steady diet of healthy greens and colorful vegetables, beans, walnuts, seeds, and fresh fruit, would the diet industry even exist? Our collective dietary ignorance is the only thing keeping that industry alive. If people understood the basic principles of nutritional excellence, they would understand that they need to eat healthfully, and by doing so they would achieve their ideal weight and never feel compelled to diet again. They wouldn't jump from one popular diet book to another looking for a quick fix. They wouldn't have to.

When you lose weight and gain it back again, you only end up fatter than before. And this regained weight is harder to lose. Even worse, all this new extra weight makes you more susceptible to disease than before you started dieting. In other words, unless you keep off the fat you lost, you're in danger.

Cycling your weight up and down takes a toll on the body. When you lose weight, you lose both fat and muscle. When you put weight back on, however, you put it back on mostly as fat. Muscle takes longer to restore—and that's only from consistent, rigorous exercise. A 1993 study examined the correlation between weight cycling and obesity in rats. Researchers restricted the caloric intake of one group of rats and kept a second group of rats on their regular diet. When they put the first group back on its regular diet, the rats in that group ended up with more body fat than the rats that were fed the same number of calories as part of their regular diet.[1] The consistency of caloric intake made for a leaner rat, while the fluctuation of calories led to a fatter rat.

The same holds true for humans. When we cut back our calories dramatically in the hopes of losing weight and then increase them once we reach our "goal weight," our lipogenic enzymes, the enzymes that store fat, shoot up. Such weight cycling is particularly harmful. It leads to more abdominal fat and visceral fat, the two types of body fat that place people at the highest risk of diabetes, heart disease, and cancer.[2]

Visceral fat is the fat under your abdominal wall. It surrounds your internal organs, engulfing your liver, intestines, kidney, pancreas, and heart with fat. Subcutaneous fat, on the other hand, is directly under your skin. It's the fat you can pinch. Visceral fat, which is deeper inside your belly, is associated with a number of serious health concerns, including high blood pressure, insulin resistance, diabetes, and heart disease. When you diet, you lose subcutaneous fat. But when you go off the diet and gain weight, you put on more visceral fat. It takes years to get rid of visceral fat. And it's almost never accomplished by crash dieting. Losing visceral fat requires a permanent commitment to healthy eating and healthy living through regular exercise.

A person's history of dieting and weight fluctuation not only leads to the accumulation of visceral fat, it may also change the type of fatty acids the body stores. Fad diets like the Paleo or Atkins diet, for instance,

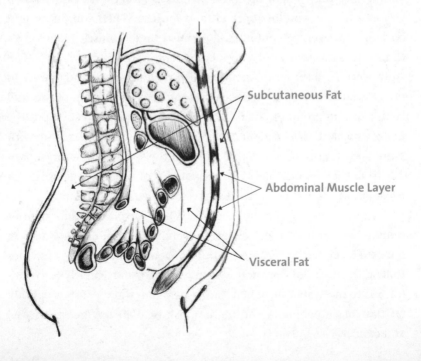

often increase the amount of saturated fats in the body's tissues, which raises your cholesterol and puts you more at risk for getting cancer.

We know this from animal experiments and human clinical trials. For example, one study put rats on a diet that caused them to lose weight and then regain the lost weight over and over. When the rats died, scientists examined the fatty acid composition of their tissues and found that the more times the rats lost and gained weight, the more saturated fats collected in their tissues. At the same time, their levels of the essential omega-3 fatty acid ALA decreased accordingly. What this means is the rats burned through their healthy essential fatty acids for energy but then couldn't replace them once they put weight back on. Without enough ALA in our adipose tissue (literally, body fat), the higher saturated fats take over, which can lead to coronary heart disease. People with a history of weight cycling demonstrate similar problems. The fluctuation in weight lowers their high-density lipoprotein (HDL) (good cholesterol), raises their low-density lipoprotein (LDL) (bad cholesterol), and increases their risk of high blood pressure and the likelihood of triggering ischemic events, such as heart attacks and strokes.[3]

Weight gain is associated with high blood pressure, especially when the weight settles in as visceral fat. Not surprisingly, then, your blood pressure increases as your body mass index increases, even when you're well within the normal BMI range for your particular height.[4]

A history of weight cycling also leads to higher fasting insulin levels. Insulin is the chief hormone responsible for increasing lipogenesis (fat storage), while simultaneously suppressing lipolysis (fat removal). For example, even as far back as 1932 a study showed that men with the longest history of weight fluctuations exhibited higher fasting insulin levels, even if their BMI was within the normal range for their height. If a man achieved a more favorable weight, his high fasting insulin level still increased, which put a tremendous amount of stress on the pancreas to balance out the increase in insulin—the first step toward diabetes. The beta cells in the pancreas that produce insulin become overworked because they're trying to keep up with the high insulin demands. Ongoing demand continuing for years causes these beta cells to fail more and more, which is when diabetes rears its ugly head.

Not only does weight cycling increase the risk of diabetes, it also lowers your good cholesterol and raises your bad cholesterol. And it raises your blood pressure in later life. A constant fluctuation in weight places significant stress on the entire cardiovascular system, increasing overall cardiovascular morbidity and premature death. Interestingly, the increased risk of cardiovascular disease isn't limited to people who are overweight. Weight cycling has an equally adverse effect in people of normal weight too.

Every time you "diet" by eating a smaller number of calories than your body would normally require to maintain a favorable weight, your body activates the enzymes that promote fat storage that can make weight loss more difficult. Some of these enzymes include fatty acid synthase, acetyl-CoA-carboxylase, ATP citrate lyase, and glucose-6-phosphate dehydrogenase. When calories are scarce, the body holds on to calories in its tissues. Activity of these enzymes inhibits the loss of fat from the body, and once these enzymes get going, it takes a long time to slow them down. Which means that once you return to eating the appropriate number or, even worse, the same number of calories you were previously eating, your body is more prone to store these calories as fat, making it more likely that you'll end up fatter than you were before you started to diet.

Self-Destruction Never Tasted So Good

Let's take a closer look at the Dukan diet, one of the most dangerous—and popular—yo-yo diets ever devised. Another rehash of the Atkins and South Beach diets, Pierre Dukan's book *The Dukan Diet* has sold more than 7 million copies since its publication in France in 2000 (it was published in the United States in 2011). The fact that this dangerous diet, cycling a person in and out of *ketosis,* became so popular demonstrates profound nutritional confusion among our population and the need for tremendous education about dieting. The first step in this diet is cutting out carbohydrates completely and eating a diet of almost all animal products.

Like Atkins, the diet lets you lose weight quickly through episodic ketosis. When you go on a very-high-protein, severely carbohydrate-restricted diet, your body becomes starved for glucose, the fuel that typically runs your body's cells and is the primary fuel for the brain. Ketosis is your body's way of making up for this lack of fuel. Since the brain and other tissues aren't getting sufficient glucose, the brain gradually accommodates to accept ketones as an emergency fuel. Ketones are a product of fat breakdown.

But ketosis doesn't come without a price. It increases acids in your bloodstream and leaches calcium from your bones. And as these acids flood your body, your body burns through stored minerals in an attempt to stop or reduce the rising acidity in your blood. Then, to purge acid from your urine, your body excretes from your system even more calcium, as well as potassium and magnesium, which creates mineral deficiencies and electrolyte imbalances that can lead to cardiac arrhythmias, or irregular heartbeats. Episodic ketosis can also lead to kidney damage.[5] High-protein, low-carbohydrate diets are also associated in scientific studies with increased risk of cardiovascular disease and premature death.[6]

More frightening is they may cause many more deaths than we know about. At the height of the Atkins craze, for instance, sudden cardiac death, which is generally caused by an irregular heartbeat, spiked dramatically in young women. Typically a danger to the middle-aged and elderly, sudden cardiac death increased by 30 percent in young women from 1990 to 2000, according to a report released by the CDC and first reported at the American Heart Association's Forty-First Annual Conference on Cardiovascular Disease Epidemiology and Prevention. This increase in death due to cardiac arrhythmia in young women is striking because it happened during a time when the overall risk of cardiac death was decreasing in our society. These unexplained anomalies could be the result of the popularity of diets that rely on high-protein ketosis. We saw similar problems related to the liquid protein fad in the 1970s.[7]

A striking example of this heightened risk of death was a medical journal report documenting the details of one of the many thousands of sudden cardiac deaths in young people, where the potential causative factors were never investigated and detailed like they were in this case:[8]

The medical journal report describes a sixteen-year-old girl who had sudden onset of cardiorespiratory arrest while at school. The investigators reported:

She had recently attempted weight loss using a low-carbohydrate/ high-protein, calorie-restricted dietary regimen that she had initiated on her own. During resuscitation, severe hypokalemia (low potassium) was noted. At postmortem examination, no other causes for the cardiac arrest were identified. Laboratory evaluation during resuscitation revealed severe hypokalemia (low potassium). Other potential causes for the condition were ruled out by parental history, autopsy findings, and postmortem toxicology evaluation.

    Bloom and Azar (published study) reported that postural hypotension can develop in subjects on low-carbohydrate diets. Using an isolated, perfused rat heart model, Russell and Taegtmeyer (published study) showed that the beating heart loses contractile function (more than 50 percent in sixty minutes) when oxidizing acetoacetate alone. Elevated levels of free fatty acids may promote both vascular thrombosis and cardiac arrhythmias. More importantly, deaths associated with other specialized diets have been reported. Our patient's sudden onset of cardiorespiratory arrest occurred without an underlying cause identified by history or on postmortem examination. Initial electrocardiogram revealed ventricular fibrillation, an unusual presenting arrhythmia in a sixteen-year-old adolescent without underlying cardiac disease or electrolyte disturbance. When considering the potential causes of these electrolyte disturbances in an otherwise healthy female adolescent, questions arise regarding the potential role of the low-carbohydrate/high-protein diet compounded by a period of inadequate caloric intake and the resultant catabolic state.

That's one serious side effect that we must consider as a strong possibility. Sudden death is obviously not the most common risk factor here. The most critical risk is the risk later in life of cancer from eating this way. However, are dieters warned about this potentially deadly risk from these popular diets? Imagine if they placed a sticker right across the front page of those books:

NEW YORK TIMES BESTSELLER. OVER 5 MILLION SOLD. BE AWARE, THIS DIET MAY CAUSE CONSTIPATION, REFLUX, BONE LOSS, AND SUDDEN CARDIAC DEATH, AND IF YOU LIVE LONG ENOUGH, CANCER.

I guess there are no authorities looking to protect the public from diet books. Yet, these authors will claim their diet is healthful and safe from a two-year study with a relatively limited number of participants. This is demonstrative of one of the problems. People do not consider long-term effects of their actions and do not realize that looking at a study that lasts for one or two years is not sufficient to ascertain risks. It would take twenty to thirty years to see pertinent findings of increased risk of cancer.

When the atomic bomb was exploded in Hiroshima and Nagasaki, Japan, in the 1940s, it took forty years to see the peak in cancer occur

from that increased radiation exposure. In general, there is a significant lag time between cause and effect when we are looking at cancer.
It takes many years of observation to state an intervention is safe.
Even increased risks of heart disease generally would take many, many
years to observe and document. Just viewing changes in lipid profile
is not adequate, as that is merely one of many risk factors and promoters of atherosclerosis. The link between high-protein diets and breast
cancer has not been investigated; however, the vast majority of the
studies examining this issue conducted over longer periods of time
show a clear link with higher meat consumption.[9] To fully appreciate
the link between diet and breast cancer, you have to examine early-
life diets in detail, not later-life diet, right before the diagnosis is made.
This is why epidemiologic studies show a strong relationship with
animal products and cancer and cohort studies on later-life adults do
not. For example, in the Shanghai Breast Cancer study, they compared
the high vegetable and soy diet pattern to women eating a higher
meat and sweet diet pattern and found a 60 percent increased risk of
breast cancer in the meat and sweet diet group.[10] The concern that
this brings up is that many of these low-carb, high-protein dieters are
younger and they are maintaining these extreme high-meat diets for
many years.

Another serious concern I have regarding the Dukan diet and other
similar diets that require you to cycle in and out of various levels of
intensity with episodic ketosis is that they cycle fat as you progress
through the different stages of the diet. You wind up losing subcutaneous fat and end up adding visceral fat to your body, where it gathers
in and around your heart—the last place you want to store any kind
of fat. These kinds of diets are dangerous to both your short-term and
long-term health.

It's important to remember, though, that you do need to keep your
weight down. Losing weight, if done correctly, is not dangerous—as

long as you keep it off. Scientific research has shown again and again that overall and abdominal obesity are strongly associated with coronary heart disease, and the severity of heart disease correlates with the number of years a person remains obese. Every year a person is obese increases the risk of death.[11]

How you lose weight is critical. Which brings us to the three basic principles of dieting:

1. If you lose weight, don't gain it back.

2. If you change your diet, change it forever.

3. The longer you remain overweight, the higher your risk of heart disease and cancer.

Don't make any changes to your diet that don't support your long-term health, and don't make any changes to your diet that you don't believe you can maintain for the rest of your life.

I have changed my diet too in recent years. In the past five years, for instance, I learned more about the disease-protective and immune-strengthening power of raw onion and cooked mushrooms, so I now eat more onions and mushrooms than I ever did before. I've never even liked raw onions as much as I do now, but you learn to like the foods you regularly eat. When you do something to benefit your long-term health, you do it for the long term. It's not dieting; it's eating for optimal health and for a more pleasurable life.

I'm lobbying for a diet change that is stable, not one that is in constant flux. Episodic periods of weight loss are unsustainable and too often result in binge eating or a gradual return to the SAD and its vicious cycle of food addiction, toxic hunger, and overeating.

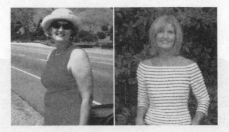

In Their Own Words

Kate lost 64 pounds and now feels "back in the land of the living." She's no longer chronically fatigued from her autoimmune disease.

BEFORE: 170 pounds

AFTER: 106 pounds

I had always considered myself a healthy eater. I stuck to organic veggies and meats, never drank colas or ate candy bars. I scrutinized the ingredients in my food. But the older I got, the worse I began to feel. I was up to 170 pounds, my total cholesterol was at 239, and my fatigue felt bottomless. I was diagnosed with pernicious anemia, a debilitating autoimmune disease. I was told that there really wasn't much that could be done other than take vitamin B_{12}, which I started immediately. Unfortunately, however, it didn't really help my fatigue.

At this point I became completely stopped in life—I couldn't work, I had zero energy, and I felt miserable all the time. No doctor at any time ever mentioned food as maybe contributing to all this. While trying to find out more about autoimmune diseases, I came across Dr. Fuhrman's *Eat to Live.* Both my husband and I started reading it immediately, and it made total sense to us. We both recognized that food was the one constant in our lives that had never really changed, despite all the different diet combinations and ratios we had tried in the past.

We both committed 100 percent to this way of eating. We've been following it for 2½ years. As a result, I went from 170 pounds to 106 pounds. My cholesterol went from 239 to 129, and my dress size went from a size 14 to a size 2! Most important, however, is my newfound energy and tremendous quality of life I now enjoy.

When people meet me for the first time, they can't believe that just a few short years earlier I was house-bound and had virtually no life at all. Now I'm actively back in the land of the living, and it's an honor to be able to share with people my story about how simple it is to get back your health and vitality by just following what Dr. Fuhrman says.

"Fast Food" Versus "Slow Food"

I call the staples of the SAD—sugar, flour, milk, and oil—*fast foods*. The term "fast food" conventionally refers to what you find at a fast-food restaurant, with its high-salt, highly processed, mass-produced meals; but I want you to categorize foods that flood the body with empty calories as fast food too. When you eat a piece of bread or chocolate cake, for instance, your body breaks down the white flour into simple glucose in the stomach, which is then absorbed into the bloodstream within minutes. Oils are processed; fast foods too. Unlike real food, they are absorbed into the bloodstream immediately. And when fats are absorbed so rapidly, the body can't burn them for energy, so they're quickly cleared from the bloodstream and stored in the body as fat. Nuts and seeds are also high-fat foods, but unlike oil and refined sweets, they take a long time to digest, and their fats are released slowly into the bloodstream. The body can then utilize them, properly, for energy.

The secret to hormonally activating your weight loss is by staying with natural whole foods and away from processed foods entirely, especially sweets and oil. For example, your body absorbs quickly the calories in white bread and apple juice, but it takes comparatively more time to absorb calories from a whole wheat berry or an apple (see Table 3).

TABLE 3. FAST CALORIES AND SLOW CALORIES

FAST CALORIES	SLOW CALORIES
Sugary drinks	Steel-cut oats
White bread	Wheat berries
Olive oil	Pistachio nuts
White potato	Adzuki beans
Apple juice	Apples

The hormones regulating fat storage and fat removal include insulin, leptin, and IGF-1. The more fat you have on your body, the more leptin it releases. Leptin is released by fatty tissue. When you start storing fat, the release of leptin tells the brain that you have plenty of energy storage and you don't need to eat. Leptin also activates receptors in the hypothalamus that suppress your appetite. So why doesn't it work? Why do people become immune to the appetite suppressive effects of leptin?

There are various reasons why, but the main one is that the body becomes resistant to leptin once its levels have been elevated too long. In other words, if you overeat and put on a few extra pounds several times in your life, your body continues to release leptin until you return to the appropriate weight. But once you spend enough of your life in a severely overweight condition, leptin just stops working, largely because the body is so overwhelmed dealing with the symptoms of toxic hunger. As a result, leptin can no longer suppress appetite.

However, the problem gets worse. Not only has your body become resistant to high levels of leptin, your leptin level also drops as you diet to lose weight, which, in turn, decreases thyroid activity and the expenditure of energy in your body's skeletal muscle. So people who have lost weight through dieting end up with a lower basal metabolic rate, which means that they burn fewer calories at rest than people at the same exact weight who didn't get to that weight by dieting. For people to start losing weight again, leptin has to be activated. More important, however, tissue sensitivity has to be reignited so the body can start to respond again to leptin and to encourage the thyroid to function normally again.

The same is true for insulin. The pancreas normally secretes very small amounts of insulin to regulate blood sugar. A healthy body needs only a small amount of insulin to move the glucose from the bloodstream into the cells of the body. The combination of a high-glycemic diet and fat on the body raises the levels of insulin higher and higher.

Stored body fat acts like a barrier to insulin function, so the pancreas responds by producing more and more of it. A high amount of insulin is harmful because excess insulin supports and drives fat storage, and it promotes angiogenesis. Angiogenesis is the growth of new blood vessels. This new blood vessel growth is necessary to feed and support the increasing mass of fatty tissue on the body. Evidence has also linked chronic hyperinsulinemia (high insulin levels) to a greater risk of cancer.[12] As your body becomes more resistant to insulin, the pancreas is forced to produce abnormally elevated levels. This overworks the insulin-producing beta cells in the pancreas, which eventually can lead to type 2 diabetes.

I've Messed Up My Body, So What Do I Do Now?

So let's assume you've spent a lifetime dieting, and in the process, you've messed up your metabolism. It's now almost impossible for you to lose weight. Don't worry. You don't have to throw in the towel. You can still lose weight, but to do so you must slow down your body's fat-storage enzymes and keep their levels down, and you must inhibit angiogenesis. You can still avoid surges in your insulin levels and insulin-like growth hormones. All you have to do is eat lots of low-glycemic plant foods such as greens, cauliflower, tomatoes, eggplant, mushroom, beans, seeds, and nuts. Such low-glycemic plant foods digest slowly and feed the body with protective nutrients.

Consuming foods that take a long time to digest is the key to re-sensitizing the body to leptin and insulin. Lucky for us, foods that take a long time to digest contain phytochemicals with angiogenesis-inhibiting effects. When you eat foods that can slowly feed your metabolism without stimulating insulin receptors, you can hormonally activate your weight loss. In other words, by giving your body better foods, it will start to naturally burn through the excess fat in your diet.

IN THEIR OWN WORDS

It took hitting rock bottom for Susan to realize that the solution to her health problems was within her grasp.

BEFORE: 350 pounds

AFTER: 140 pounds

As another birthday approached, I found myself at a whopping 350 pounds. I was diabetic, hypertensive, and very depressed. Ironically, I only had to look as far as my own bookshelf to find a prescription to better health, *Eat to Live* by Dr. Fuhrman. It was signed: "Wishing you all good health and much happiness always, Joel Fuhrman."

I remember my first meeting with Dr. Fuhrman. He let me know in no uncertain terms that my current lifestyle was going to lead to disease and an early grave. But I continued my destructive course, and continued to live to eat.

Through the years, I tried many different weight-loss programs and found only temporary successes. In 2005, at 350 pounds, I had a lapband procedure, probably one of the worst decisions I have ever made. The restrictive band made it almost impossible to eat a healthy, well-balanced diet. In fact, it made it most comfortable to eat foods that were literally sugar-coated. Eventually, I had the band opened to its fullest extent and continued trying new fads.

I finally took *Eat to Live* off the shelf, knowing that in my hands was my greatest hope for a healthy future. Since then, I have lost 210 pounds. I now enjoy physical activities. On my fiftieth birthday, I climbed a mountain in Woodstock, New York—and then enjoyed a meal of kale, roasted beets, and beans! I ride my bicycle with my son, too. Our last trek was fourteen miles, much of it uphill. My husband and I traveled to Paris to visit our daughter, a vacation I never would have dreamed of because of the expense and humiliation of buying two airplane seats for one obese person.

I love telling my story. This diet style is easy to follow. I rarely weigh or measure any food. I don't feel like I'm on a diet—because if I'm hungry, I eat.

The nutritarian diet style is *not* a burden—being morbidly obese and sidelined from your own life *is*!

Certain foods downregulate fat-storage hormones because they're packed with angiogenesis inhibitors and hormone-inhibiting phytochemicals (Table 4). Angiogenesis inhibition prevents the growth of new blood vessels, which is needed to expand your fat deposits. By inhibiting the growth of blood vessels, you prevent your body from getting fat. At the same time, this also helps you lose fat over time. The body literally can rebuild itself, and its architecture is shaped by the foods you choose to eat.

When you consume plant foods that are high in nutrients and phytochemicals, your body will start to repair itself via multiple mechanisms. For example, parsley, arugula, scallions, and watercress are simple low-calorie foods that contain hundreds of body-fixing nutrients that oppose body fat accumulation. They douse us with nutrients, with very few calories in the process. They haven't had the phytochemicals bred out of them through commercial propagation and food engineering, like white potatoes and corn have. Because of their high content of phytochemicals, these and other natural foods encourage fat loss and make possible a favorable weight for the rest of your life. Eating the right foods helps people resolve their lifelong struggle with their weight, while simultaneously protecting against cancer.

In addition to reducing hormones that facilitate fat storage, phytochemicals also help restore your body's normal fat-burning metabolism. And phytochemicals can reduce the amount of fatty tissue on your body by inducing *apoptosis,* or the killing off of existing fat cells.

Polyphenols, a complex mixture of many plant pigments, do the same thing. When you consume natural foods that contain phytochemicals and polyphenols, you can decrease the number of bacteria in your gut that promote fat storage and increase the number that encourage a slim body.[13] A high consumption of polyphenols leads to an increase in bacteria that interfere with the breakdown of carbohydrates into simple sugars. Foods high in polyphenols lower blood glucose levels and enhance insulin sensitivity. They keep you slim. Beans, greens, tomatoes, seeds, and berries contain loads and loads of phytochemicals *and* polyphenols that restore a healthy fat metabolism and oppose body fat storage.

Furthermore, a high consumption of colorful plant foods creates an abundance of bifidobacteria and lactobacilli, as well as many other microorganisms that benefit our health and our weight. A diet of refined foods or heavy in meat supports the growth of bacteria that release inflammatory compounds, increase insulin resistance, and promote fat storage and atherosclerosis.[14] This means that it isn't primarily *how much* you eat that makes you overweight, but *what* you eat. This, in a nutshell, is the most important reason that so many people are overweight and can't lose weight. It's not enough to eat less; you have to eat differently.

TABLE 4. FAT-REDUCING PHYTOCHEMICALS

Alkaloids	Genistein
Anthocyanins	Phenolic acids
Epigallocatechin	Resveratrol
Flavonoids	Stilbenoids

In addition to their low caloric content, high-nutrient plant foods have anti-obesity and anti-diabetic effects (see Table 5, opposite).[15] Almost everybody thinks that dieting is still about counting calories, exercising more, and having the willpower to eat less food. And then they're told that if they don't have the willpower to do these things, they need to have surgery to remove three-quarters of their stomach. This conventional way of thinking is the problem, not the solution.

The same beneficial hormonal parameters that facilitate the reduction of body fat also protect against cancer, especially prostate and breast cancer. In other words, eating to prevent cancer also prevents fat storage in the body and vice versa.

More and more we're discovering multiple mechanisms that lead to weight gain. And in the process, we learn the secret to permanent weight loss. Eating the right foods is the secret to removing the common obstacles to weight reduction. When you eat right, you restore the proper biochemical mix of body hormones, gut bacteria, and fuel cellular repair to make the body function right. The balance of favorable microorganisms in your digestive tract is an often overlooked factor that helps keep your weight down.

TABLE 5. FOODS THAT FIGHT FAT

Artichokes	Mushrooms
Arugula	Parsley
Black raspberries	Pomegranates
Blueberries	Pumpkin seeds
Broccoli	Red onions
Cauliflower	Scallions
Collards	Soybeans (edamame)
Eggplant	Strawberries
Garlic	Tomatoes
Green tea	Turmeric
Kale	Watercress
Lettuce	

The list in Table 5 is only partial. How many of the items in the table do you eat in your regular diet? I try to eat as many of them as I can every day. I add them to my breakfast oats or fruit, I add them to my lunch salad or soup, and I eat them as part of my dinner. In other words, I might add chopped raw scallions to my hot soup and raw onions, watercress, and tomatoes to my mushroom bean burger.

Eat hefty portions of the foods that fight fat, and you won't be dieting. You'll be eating for health and longevity with plenty of great-tasting, satisfying foods—which just happen to interfere with fat storage and facilitate weight reduction. You don't have to weigh portions and count calories because a bigger portion of these foods is better than a smaller one. Instead of eating less food, then, eat three substantially sized meals a day—of the right kinds of food.

Green Makes You Lean

Once you get back to eating real food, you don't have to diet to become slim. You can eat as much as you want. You don't have to skimp, you can eat in abundance, and your taste will grow to prefer the healthy food that makes your body feel so good. It takes time for your body and mind to adjust to this, but it *does* happen.

You have to change the way you eat permanently, however, and you have to remember that it takes time for enzymes to return to a normal state. Be patient and remember that there's no such thing as a quick fix.

At the beginning, you have to start somewhere, and the place to start is with salads. The first foods you eat at a meal influence how much you eat and what you eat. Make salad the main dish; make it big, and make it first. This is the simplest and most effective way to prevent overeating and to make sure you never have a weight problem. The only thing you have to remember is to not stuff yourself until you're uncomfortable. You shouldn't be aware of your stomach. How does your liver feel today? Are you a little uncomfortable in your pancreas or adrenals? The point here is that we don't feel that these organs even exist. You shouldn't be aware of your internal organs, including your stomach. So you shouldn't eat until your stomach feels uncomfortable.

Recently I had some old friends over for dinner. We didn't prepare anything in advance; when they arrived, we all made the food together. Some chopped the watercress, scallions, and onion. Some chopped the lettuce and other greens. Others sliced tomatoes and strawberries, one peeled a few oranges, and I made salad dressing by blending oranges, lemon, blood orange vinegar, toasted sesame seeds, and some raw cashew pieces. We had a great salad that included strawberries, onions, scallions, watercress, radicchio, baby lettuces, and frisée lettuce. It was super delicious and super healthy. Then we had some homemade mixed-bean chili with shiitake mushrooms, and some creamy, sweet ice cream for dessert made from blending frozen mango with a young coconut.

When you eat for optimal health, you can eat as much as you want, feel satisfied, and intellectually and emotionally feel great about what you eat. You restore your metabolism to normal, inhibit fat storage in your body, become lean, and cancer-proof your body simultaneously.

Let's End the Insanity

About half of all Americans are on a diet. The other half have just given up dieting and are currently on a binge. Collectively, we're overweight, sickly, and struggling. We've made it socially acceptable to be a nation of food addicts, forfeiting our health via a toxic diet. In fact, people in the United States are ostracized if they don't take part in self-destructive habits. Instead of supporting, reinforcing, and applauding those who take good care of their health with superior nutrition and regular exercise, people call them "health nuts" and criticize them for being extreme. It's normal to continually stoke the body with addictive substances—alcohol, addictive and unhealthy foods, and prescription drugs.

Now is the time to acknowledge, understand, and end this insanity.

We've made it socially unacceptable in the United States to smoke cigarettes. Now we have to make it socially unacceptable to drink soft drinks and to eat candy and fried foods. These are simply self-destructive and irresponsible behaviors, just like smoking, snorting cocaine, and getting drunk. We as a nation have to stop dieting and looking for a magic fix. We need to accept the fact that all of us are individually responsible for putting in our mouths high-quality, nourishing food. Eat little salt and very little animal products, if you eat them at all. Eat mostly vegetables, beans, fruits, onions, and mushrooms. Don't eat sweets or anything white. Get off your butt and be active, exercising every day. Stop dieting, go live, be productive, and let's heal the world.

To paraphrase President John F. Kennedy, "It's not what your diet can do for you, it's what your diet can do for your country." (Or something like that.) Our country is in the pits, and it's not getting out until we become a healthier, more productive population with fewer medical costs. We can never afford to pay for so many sick individuals, given the tremendous medical costs involved and especially within the context of our litigious society.

We are paying for this fast-food genocide with our shared tax dollars. When people eat themselves into coronary bypass surgery or wind up in nursing homes, we pay for it with our tax dollars and national debt. Our sickly population destroys our economy and weakens our businesses; our industries can't compete in the world market because of such high medical expenditures.

More than 85 percent of U.S. workers are overweight or obese, and the resulting and chronic diseases have lowered productivity, increased the number of sick days, and increased healthcare costs, among other expenses. These expenses are rising geometrically, outstripping other costs, and making our products noncompetitive in the world marketplace. Fast food, soda and energy drinks, snack foods, and specialty beverages are now commonplace. We practice "sickcare," not "healthcare," and we can't afford sickcare now, which is 20 percent of our gross domestic product and rising. How are we going to afford this as costs rise even higher? According to the American Heart Association, the costs of treating heart disease and stroke are expected to triple in the next twenty years to $818 billion per year.

We simply have an unacceptable level of health problems and health tragedies, reducing the quality of our lives. Plus, we need a healthier population to improve our economy, and we need a population eating healthier foods to benefit our environment, too. Obviously, eating right will do all: It will protect us and also help our country and our planet. Eating right is the right thing to do.

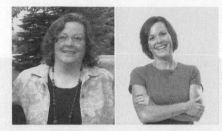

first time in my adult life I was free from the "dieting mentality" that failed me miserably.

Change the Mind and the Body Will Follow

Intrigued by the experiences of others, Emily began interviewing successful nutritarians for my blog and gleaned invaluable nuggets of truth from many other real-life success stories. With my guidance and from these experiences and observations, Emily compiled twelve vital tips for losing weight—and keeping it off— the nutritarian way.

1. It Takes Commitment.

Success has nothing to do with economic status, nationality, education, social standing, professional training, career choice, a stable upbringing, or even support from loved ones. Success is a direct result of thoroughly studying, understanding, and assimilating the science behind Dr. Fuhrman's nutritional recommendations—and then making the decision to tenaciously earn your health back, no matter what. Success is having both feet in at all times, not "trying" to eat high-nutrient foods during the week and indulging on the weekends, or eating for health only when it's convenient. Trying only leaves the door cracked open to indulging on a whim. All who have succeeded made the firm decision to commit 100 percent.

2. Perspective Determines Outcome.

Those who succeed with the nutritarian approach view it as an opportunity to "earn" health back. This perspective enables a person to get past toxic cravings to thoroughly enjoy great-tasting foods, in their natural state. Conversely, those who repeatedly fail have the mind-set of dieting. They view the nutritarian approach as just another diet designed only to lose weight and subsequently focus on restriction and deprivation. This mentality invites self-pity and cheating, which doesn't allow your taste buds to change or let you break free of the vicious cycle of toxic addiction.

3. Change a Mistaken Identity.

People become what they believe to be true about themselves and what they repeatedly tell others. If people believe they are failures, they will fail. If they tell everyone that they are a compulsive overeater, they will compulsively over-eat in times of stress. It's vitally important to declare and believe in an identity congruent with who you want to be. If you want to be a nutritarian—someone who eats high-nutrient foods to meet the body's biological needs for optimal nutrition—then declare it! Make it your identity. Where the mind goes, the body will follow.

4. Ditch the Wagon.
The wagon mentality and dieting go hand in hand. "I fell off the wagon" basi-cally translates into, "I blew it so I might as well eat anything I want now." Eat-ing for optimal health is a lifetime endeavor of making wise choices each and every day. Slipups do happen from time to time, but never allow a slipup to turn into an excuse to wallow in disappointment, self-pity, and false guilt that could potentially lead to a full-fledged binge.

5. Avoid the Moderation Myth.
When it comes to toxic foods, there's no such thing as eating in moderation. Taking just one bite of an addictive food can be just as dangerous as smok-ing one cigarette for a former nicotine addict. Don't believe the moderation myth that you might hear from physicians, counselors, ministers, friends, co-workers, or relatives. The truth is that just one bite of an addictive food can do great harm. It's much easier to keep addictive cravings extinguished than to be continually fighting obsessive compulsions, because it only takes a tiny spark to ignite them.

6. There Are No Shortcuts.
Everyone has to cross the threshold of withdrawal from toxic foods, which, for most people, is no fun. Detoxification (or toxic hunger) can be unpleasant. You might experience headaches, nausea, weakness, fatigue, shakiness, and irrita-bility that can last up to several days. But once the symptoms have resolved, and if you no longer consume toxic foods, the symptoms don't return. Salt is a particularly tough habit to kick, but once the addiction to salt is gone, your taste buds change, and the subtle flavors of fruits and vegetables in their natu-ral state become highly enjoyable.

7. Tomorrow Never Comes.

Waiting until after the holidays or a special occasion to begin eating for health is a bad idea. Telling yourself you'll "start tomorrow" is a lie. There's always another celebration or family event. After Thanksgiving, Hanukkah, and Christmas comes the Super Bowl, followed by Valentine's Day, Passover, Easter, Mother's Day, graduation parties, multiple birthday parties, a wedding or two, a Father's Day cookout, summer barbecues and picnics, county fairs, fall festivals, Halloween, and then the year-end holidays all over again. You must make the firm decision to eat for health each day and hold fast to that commitment no matter what the calendar says.

8. The Refrigerator Is Never the Solution.

Eating is never a solution to any problem. Ever. Emotional health is never achieved via the refrigerator, cupboard, or drive-thru window. Life is full of ups and downs, joys and sorrows, pleasures and pains; that's why our lives are interesting and, ultimately, fulfilling. Address emotional issues by talking to a professional counselor or a trusted family member or friend, or join a support group. Addictive foods and drugs are never the solution.

9. Abstinence Is Important.

The purpose of an established boundary is to keep you safe. In that safe place you'll find freedom from addiction and disease. Food addiction can be as serious as alcoholism and drug addiction. It destroys lives. A commitment to abstain from all processed foods and junk food is often needed. Abstinence is radical, but it produces the best results. That means if you are a food addict and have cravings and trigger foods that drive unhealthful eating, then you need to abstain from these known triggers. The most effective way to beat the addictive drive to overconsume alcohol, drugs, or sweets is abstinence for at least a few months. Many people are highly addicted to sweets and refined carbohydrates and need to abstain.

10. Have a Plan and Stick to It.

Getting out and staying out of food addiction isn't that hard per se, but you must be vigilant and persistent at all times. When I finally committed to follow Dr. Fuhrman's nutritarian approach, I typed out his Six-Week Plan, printed off several copies, and had them laminated. I put one in my purse and another in my car; I posted one on my bathroom mirror and another on the refrigerator. I even attached one to my ironing board! That tangible plan made all the decisions for me. Three months later I was 40 pounds lighter, and my blood pressure, fasting blood sugar levels, and lipid profile were all normal; and even more importantly, the overwhelming cravings for toxic foods were completely gone!

11. Be Prepared At All Times.
Plan ahead and always have food prepared in advance. Your health destiny is your responsibility, so be prepared at all times. Unlike junk food dieting, no factory-prepared meals will be delivered to your doorstep. Keep your refrigerator well stocked with freshly cleaned vegetables, fruits, and cooked bean soups for quick meals. Never wait until the refrigerator is empty to plan and prepare more food. Once you establish a routine of preparation, it will become second nature—but in the beginning, you have to make this habit a top priority to develop it.

12. Never Give Up.
Hard times happen. When life is turned upside down, it takes everything within yourself to muster the strength to keep going in the direction of health. But even when you have challenging days, stay committed to making wise food choices as best as you can. There is never a valid excuse to quit. As Dr. Fuhrman states: "It will take strength, it will take effort, but the pleasures and rewards that you'll get from a healthy life will be priceless."

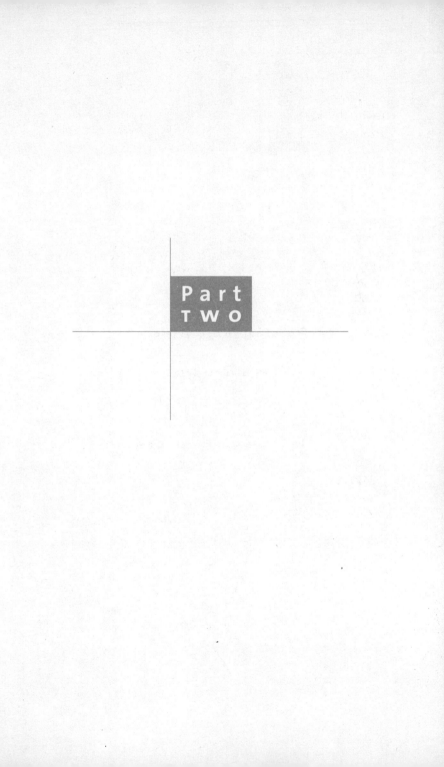

Part
TWO

CHAPTER FOUR

The Power of Real Food

You will be free from the overwhelming cravings of disease-promoting foods.

You will enjoy life without feeling miserably bloated, tired, and depressed.

You will wake up in the morning feeling refreshed and happy to be alive.

You will get to live your life free of unnecessary medical bills and pharmaceuticals.

You will be free from type 2 diabetes and heart disease.

You will save astronomical amounts of money that we might otherwise spend on unhealthy foods, medical bills, and medications.

You can live without fear of having a heart attack.

You can avoid bypass surgery and its complications.

You can sit in an airplane seat and not be encumbered by rolls of fat.

You can buckle that seat belt without the addition of an extension belt.

Embrace the opportunity to be a nutritarian by choosing high-nutrient foods and healthy habits. You'll experience the most pleasure, satisfaction, and quality out of life knowing that you're supporting, not destroying, your health as you enjoy eating!

The Healing Power Is Yours

Why doesn't everyone know that they can reverse high blood pressure and coronary artery disease with the right food and diet style? Why don't doctors tell their patients that they can eliminate the need for medications, angioplasty, and bypass surgery by changing the way they eat? A nutritarian diet is so dramatically effective that every doctor should inform their patients of this option.

Superior nutrition is the most powerful medicine; pharmacological medicine is comparably close to worthless—especially because a drug prescription gives people tacit permission to continue the same disease-causing diet that caused their problems in the first place. Have diabetes but still want that donut? No problem. Take another injection of insulin or up your dose of oral medication and enjoy yourself. In the meantime, the diabetes continues to advance unabated and under the same general conditions that enabled its development.

Everyone deserves to know that he or she can choose *not* to succumb to heart attacks and strokes. Everyone deserves to know that cancer is *not* a product of bad luck, predominantly genetic, or triggered by some mysterious, unknown cause and that nutritional science can dramatically protect us from developing cancer. Advancements in nutritional science can enable everyone to enjoy longer, better, and more fulfilling lives—entirely free from medical dependence and physical and mental disability.

People deserve to know exactly what they need to do to protect against disease. Drugs can't do this; only nutritional excellence can. Excellent nutrition is the best medicine. Who would want to be in a nursing home with half their body paralyzed if they could avoid it? Who would choose dementia over emotional and intellectual wellness through old age? Who would choose an early death over a long life? No one!

No one needs to worry about heart attack or stroke. Even common cancers would be rare in a society that followed a nutritarian diet. The standard American diet dramatically reduces the average lifespan and drastically diminishes quality of life and vigor for living. It also leads to premature aging and the onset of chronic disease, which need not happen when you eat for health.

Our body is composed of the substances we eat. We build tissue, repair tissue, maintain our health, and reach our human potential on the basis of the quality of the foods we eat. How could this fact be denied? People do not sufficiently appreciate or even recognize the importance and magnificence of this simple concept. For example, studies determined that poor nutrition early in life predisposes people to antisocial and criminal behavior and lowers intelligence.[1]

Violence, prison, and diminished intelligence are consequences that we don't currently associate with an unhealthy diet. We have been conditioned to believe that the source of one's calories doesn't matter.

Then, as we get older, too many of us develop high blood pressure, high cholesterol, diabetes, and heart disease. These serious problems, we are told, are inevitable consequences of aging. And we blindly accept that fact. All we can do is take drugs and let doctors perform palliative procedures that make our "numbers" look better, while our health continues to deteriorate every year. When we require drugs to camouflage our medical problems, we are not well. Yet, these chronic conditions never need to happen and are reversible if we do something about them before we drop dead. What follows is what we all need to know exceedingly well: Nutrition 101.

Macronutrients and Micronutrients

Food supplies us with both calories (energy) and nutrients. The four macronutrients are fat, carbohydrate, protein, and water. Though free of calories, water is considered a macronutrient because the body requires such a relatively large quantity—a "macro" amount—of it for survival. All the foods we eat contain some combination of the three calorie-containing macronutrients. Macronutrients are how we get the calories we need for energy and growth. If you eat too many macronutrients, you're abusing calories, which leads to weight gain, chronic medical conditions, and premature death. However, there remains a broad acceptable range in the proportion of macronutrients you consume, as long as you're not eating too many calories. In other words, a well-designed diet with 15 percent of calories from fat could be healthy as well as a diet with 30 percent of calories from fat.

To lose weight and improve your health, you need to eat less fat, less carbohydrate, and less protein. Which means you have to reduce your total caloric intake. But the secret is not to count calories to reduce calories—or to worry about where you're getting the calories from. This process never works. Trying to micromanage the precise amount of each caloric source misses the most critical issue in human nutrition: meeting your macronutrient needs without excess, while getting sufficient micronutrients in the process.

Micronutrients—such as vitamins, minerals, fibers, and phytochemicals—supply critical chemical factors for life and health in small quantities and don't contain calories. Vitamins are organic compounds required by animals that cannot be synthesized by the body but are nevertheless necessary for normal cell function. Vitamins are classified as either water-soluble or fat-soluble. Of the thirteen currently recognized vitamins, four are fat-soluble (vitamins A, D, E, and K) and nine are water-soluble (eight B vitamins and vitamin C). Water-soluble vitamins dissolve easily in water and in general are readily excreted from the body. Because the body has a hard time storing these vitamins, it requires a more consistent intake of them.

The human body requires at least sixteen minerals. Minerals are tricky, though, because their range of optimal benefit is narrow. Too much or too little iron, selenium, copper, or zinc, for instance, can be unhealthy, even harmful. Too much red meat can introduce into your system a potentially harmful amount of iron and copper,[2] though in general the SAD is severely deficient in most vital micronutrients. Determining the optimal level of mineral intake, then, is crucial.

The safest and surest way to get adequate vitamins and minerals is to eat natural plant foods, including nutrient-rich colorful vegetation such as broccoli, scallions, and tomatoes. When anthropologist Katharine Milton tracked the eating habits of four different species of monkeys, she found that each species consumed about ten times the recommended daily amount of vitamin C and about four times the recommended daily amount of magnesium and potassium. They also consumed much higher amounts of the essential omega-3 fatty acid ALA.[3] Nonhuman primates eat a diet tremendously rich in disease-fighting micronutrients and phytochemicals from a diversity of plants, which is the primary cause of their longevity and robust health. Our need for nutrients and our digestive systems are no different physiologically from those of the great apes; we too need a diet full of nutrient-rich, colorful vegetation to approach the optimal level of nutrition our bodies need. The amount of colorful vegetation most people in the United States consume is dismally low, and this lack is responsible for the exploding rates of cancer and autoimmune diseases during the past century.

A nutritarian diet is also characterized by the avoidance of sugar and sweeteners, white flour, refined oils, and all kinds of processed foods—foods that are ill-adapted to the design of our species and are linked to cancer. With modern refrigeration and transportation we now have year-round access to the healthiest and most nutrient-rich foods on the planet. We also have the best opportunity, like never before, to achieve and maintain optimal health. Over the past fifty years, more than ten thousand studies have shown the benefits of consuming natural, nutrient-rich plant foods. Here are a few critical points worth considering:

- Plants contain three classes of micronutrients that are critical to our health: vitamins, minerals, and phytochemicals. These nutrients are essential for a highly effective immune system and protection from the common ravages of aging.

- Colorful vegetables, beans, and fruits have a low caloric density, allowing us to eat more food. With so many high-nutrient foods permitted in a relatively unlimited quantity, it's easy to eat to fulfillment and still lose weight and maintain an ideal weight—without the need to count calories or restrict portions.

• Increasing micronutrient intake through eating a diet of natural foods reduces appetite and cravings and restores normal hunger signals, allowing you to maintain a lean body mass while simultaneously conferring an assortment of protective health benefits that defy the aging process.

Eating foods that are rich in micronutrients is essential to good health. Foods that are naturally rich in micronutrients are also naturally rich in fiber and water. They are also naturally low in calories. By eating more nutrient-rich foods and fewer high-calorie, low-nutrient foods, we naturally lose weight and optimize our health. And the more high-nutrient food we consume, the less low-nutrient food we crave. The less low-nutrient food we crave, the more weight we lose and the healthier we become. It's that simple.

Phytochemicals: The Secret to Longevity

Essential for normal immune function and disease resistance, phytochemicals are complex chemical compounds that occur naturally in plants (*phyto* comes from the Greek word for "plant"—*phyton*). Phytochemicals support self-reparative mechanisms in cells and enable the body's defense system to work against waste products, such as free radicals and advanced glycation end products. There are more than ten thousand plant phytochemicals with the potential to prevent various diseases, including cancer. Lycopene in tomatoes, for instance, and lutein and zeaxanthin in green and yellow vegetables inhibit macular degeneration and cataracts in the eyes.[4]

Some of the most important phytochemicals are *isothiocyanates* (ITCs), which are potent immune-strengthening and vital cancer-fighting agents. ITCs have been found to fight inflammation, inhibit angiogenesis, increase the body's natural detoxification enzymes, and help kill off cancerous cells, to name just a few health benefits.[5] Plus, these antiangiogenic effects do not just block the growth

Glucosinolates When Mixed with
Myrosinase Generates ITCs

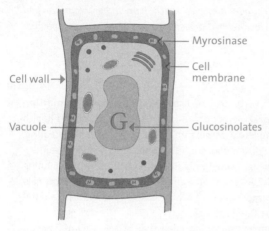

of tumors and cancers; they also inhibit the accumulation of fat on the body.

The cruciferous vegetables (Table 6) are unique because of their content of the organic compounds called *glucosinolates*. The glucosinolates in cruciferous vegetables are converted into ITCs when the plant cell wall is broken down—by chewing, juicing, chopping, or blending. The myrosinase enzyme is housed in the cell wall, which catalyzes the conversion of glucosinolates to ITCs when cells are broken. The point is, the better you chew the vegetables, the more ITCs are formed.

TABLE 6. CRUCIFEROUS VEGETABLES

Arugula	Horseradish
Bok choy	Kale
Broccoli	Kohlrabi
Broccolini	Mustard greens
Broccoli rabe	Radish
Brussels sprouts	Red cabbage
Cabbage	Rutabaga
Cauliflower	Turnip greens
Chinese cabbage	Turnips
Collards	Watercress

IN THEIR OWN WORDS

McKinley adopted a nutritarian lifestyle, which helped her identify—and overcome—the root of her food-related anxiety. She now feels free to enjoy her life in full.

BEFORE: 160 pounds

AFTER: 125 pounds

Though I'm only twenty-six years old, I can firmly say that becoming a nutritarian has given me my life back. Before discovering Dr. Fuhrman and his health equation, my life was completely dominated by a fear of food, binge eating, cyclical dieting, weight gain, and poor physical condition. I found myself trying diets one by one, my weight constantly fluctuating, my cravings spiraling totally out of control, my feelings of shame and failure immense and unspeakably devastating. I literally spent years of my life walking around with a notebook recording every single thing I ate.

I came across Dr. Fuhrman's nutritarian diet style at a very painful period in my life. I had lost two pregnancies in a relatively short period of time and my mother was starting to show signs of kidney damage following several years of a high-protein diet to control diabetes.

At first, I was very skeptical, but as I continued to read, my heart began to race. Here was a plan backed by literally thousands of research papers, and the people who followed it were reversing many types of conditions—from autoimmune disorders to diabetes to heart disease.

For the first time in my life, I haven't lost hope and I haven't given up. I no longer suffer from fear, food restriction, and despair. Physically, I'm no longer troubled by the frightening pain around the varicose veins in my right knee and calf, the chronic anemia, the restless leg syndrome, the frequent insomnia, the periods of IBS-like symptoms, the severe mood swings and depression, the migraines, poor complexion, dry mouth, and chapped skin. My life feels normal now, and balanced. I now enjoy a loving relationship with my body that is founded in a thorough understanding that wellness is almost exclusively the result of nutrition and lifestyle.

But my greatest joy is this: After seeing my sustained enthusiasm and conviction for the nutritarian lifestyle, my mom, a fifteen-plus-year diabetic and a Hoosier girl who loved typical Midwest fare, started Dr. Fuhrman's knowledge-based program early last fall. She's now very happy living the nutritarian life. Together, we're learning and working with the goal that she will be off all medications by the end of this year!

Eating cruciferous vegetables produces measurable ITCs in breast tissue, and observational studies have shown that women who eat more cruciferous vegetables are less likely to be diagnosed with breast cancer.[6] A recent study of Chinese women, for example, found that those who regularly ate one serving each day of cruciferous vegetables reduced their risk of breast cancer by 50 percent.[7] Similarly, a European study found that women who consumed cruciferous vegetables at least once a week decreased their risk of breast cancer by 17 percent.[8]

Another study tracked the cruciferous vegetable intake of Chinese women with breast cancer for the first three years after their initial diagnosis and then followed them for another five years. The more cruciferous vegetables the women ate, the less likely they were to experience breast cancer recurrence or to die from breast cancer. Women who ate higher amounts of these vegetables exhibited a 62 percent decrease in risk.[9]

Such data are supported further by the Women's Healthy Eating and Living (WHEL) study. Breast cancer survivors who reported higher than a median intake of cruciferous vegetables, and were in the top third of total vegetable intake, showed a 52 percent reduced risk of recurrence. This result is especially powerful considering that average intakes were quite low—only 3.1 and 0.5 servings a day of total and cruciferous vegetables, respectively.[10]

Now is the best time to eat cruciferous vegetables
every single day.

Green cruciferous vegetables aren't alone, though. Plant foods of all colors are rich in various disease-protective phytochemicals. *Carotenoids* are a family of more than six hundred pigmented phytochemicals including alpha-carotene, beta-carotene, lycopene, lutein, zeaxanthin, and astaxanthin. Abundant in green and yellow-orange vegetables and fruits, carotenoids help to defend the body's tissues against oxidative damage from free radicals, a known contributor to chronic disease and an accepted mechanism of aging.

A well-nourished body houses a high-functioning immune system, and the same immune cells that protect us against bacteria and viruses also protect us against cancer. Vegetables, particularly cruciferous vegetables, are the most nutrient-rich foods available. But, as you'll see, they aren't the *only* nutrient-rich foods available. As a nutritarian, you'll not only eat plenty of green vegetables, but you'll also eat a ton of other superfoods that work together to make the body cancer proof.

G-BOMBS

G	B	O	M	B	S
Greens	Beans	Onions	Mushrooms	Berries	Seeds

As I describe in my book *Super Immunity,* G-BOMBS (Greens, Beans, Onions, Mushrooms, Berries, and Seeds) are the foods with the most powerful immune-boosting and anticancer effects. These foods help to prevent the cancerous transformation of normal cells and keep the body armed and ready to attack any precancerous or cancerous cells that may arise.

G: Greens
All greens, even lettuce, have powerful antioxidant and anticancer effects.[11] Green vegetables contain compounds with anticancer substances that protect blood vessels; they also promote healthy vision and reduce the risk of developing diabetes.[12] Lettuce contains a number of antioxidant phytochemicals, including beta-carotene, lutein, zeaxanthin, vitamin C, caffeic acid, quercetin, and anthocyanins[13]—all of which contribute to observed decreases in the risk of developing cancer and cardiovascular disease. In other words, eating a huge salad as your main dish at least once a day is good for your health.

Meta-analyses of observational studies by the American Institute for Cancer Research have found that consumption of raw vegetables had dose-dependent protective effects against oral and esophageal cancers. In similar analyses, both salad greens and raw vegetables decreased the risk of stomach cancer. A daily 50-gram serving of salad greens (about 2 cups), for instance, was estimated to produce a 57 percent reduction in risk.[14] Several observational studies have also reported a reduced risk of breast cancer with the increased consumption of raw vegetables.[15] The anticancer benefits are more powerful and consistent for raw compared with cooked vegetables in the studies.

Other studies corroborate that the consumption of salads and raw vegetables reduced the risk of cancers and cardiovascular disease. A high consumption was linked to a 41 percent reduction in the risk of heart attack and a 50 percent reduced risk of stroke.[16]

Not only does eating lettuce and other raw salad vegetables protect your health; it also helps you lose and control your weight. When women were given salads as a first course, or with a main course, they ate fewer calories during the rest of the meal.[17]

B: Beans

Beans (plus lentils and other legumes) act as anti-diabetes and weight-loss foods because the body digests them slowly, which stabilizes blood sugar levels, reducing hunger and caloric drive and helping to prevent food cravings.[18] Beans are unique foods because of their very high levels of fiber and resistant starch—that is, carbohydrates that aren't broken down by digestive enzymes. The fiber and resistant starch in beans reduce the total number of calories absorbed from beans (about a third of the carbohydrate calories contained in beans may not get absorbed, but more studies are needed to accurately quantify this amount).[19] I have taught for years that beans are nutritionally superior to whole grains and should be the preferred starch source for diabetics; I often call my dietary recommendations for diabetics "the greens and beans diet." A new study published by the research group of Dr. David Jenkins, who originally developed the concept of the glycemic index (discussed more in the next chapter), has confirmed the advantages of beans over whole grains, especially for diabetics and people trying to lose weight.[20] When diabetics switch from white flour, sugar, and white rice to whole grains in their diet, they experience significant health benefits. Plus, when they switch from white potatoes to whole grains, they experience significant glycemic and other benefits, since whole grains have a comparatively lower glycemic index and more fiber than white potatoes.[21] But when diabetics rely on beans as their primary carbohydrate source instead of whole grains, they see even *more* benefits, in lower blood glucose levels—dramatic evidence of the nutritional superiority of beans as a carbohydrate source. In Jenkins's study, the group eating more beans and fewer whole grains also saw more of a reduction in cholesterol levels. Beans are rich in minerals and fiber, especially soluble fiber, and low in glycemic load—characteristics that have blood pressure–lowering effects.[22] People who eat more beans tend to have lower blood pressure in addition to higher levels of fiber and minerals, lower body weight, and a smaller waist circumference.[23] The decrease in blood pressure in the bean group significantly improved their calculated Framingham risk score, an estimate of heart disease risk over the following ten years. This is an extremely important point, since most diabetics die of heart disease or stroke.

Beans also have considerable anticancer effects. The resistant starches in beans are converted by healthy gut bacteria into fatty acids that help to prevent colon cancer. Eating beans, peas, or lentils more than twice a week has been found to decrease colon cancer risk by 50 percent.[24] Beans not only protect the colon against cancer, but a high bean intake is also associated with a decreased risk of esophageal, stomach, kidney, and breast cancers.[25] Plus, a recent analysis of ten scientific studies has shown that the higher your fiber intake, the lower your risk of breast cancer.[26]

O: Onions

The *Allium* genus of vegetables includes onions, garlic, leeks, chives, shallots, and scallions. They not only add great flavor to meals, they have beneficial effects on the cardiovascular and immune systems, as well as anti-diabetic and anticancer effects.[27] These vegetables are known for their characteristic (and eye-irritating) organosulfur compounds, which slow tumor growth and kill cancer cells. Eating onions and garlic frequently is associated with a reduced risk of cancers of the digestive tract. These vegetables also contain high concentrations of anti-inflammatory flavonoid antioxidants that contribute to their anticancer properties.[28]

Epidemiological studies have found that increased consumption of allium vegetables is associated with a decreased risk of several cancers. For example, one large European study found striking risk reductions in oral, esophageal, colorectal, laryngeal, breast, ovarian, and prostate cancers in the participants who consumed the greatest quantities of onions or garlic—an amazing 55 to 85 percent reduction![29]

Similar to the myrosinase enzyme in cruciferous vegetables, the alliinase enzyme in allium vegetables catalyzes the reaction that makes cancer-fighting organosulfur compounds, which are produced when the cell walls of the vegetables are broken down by chopping, crushing, or chewing.

In scientific studies, organosulfur compounds have been shown to prevent the development of cancers by detoxifying carcinogens and halting cancer cell growth. These garlic and onion phytochemicals are also antiangiogenic, which means that they can prevent tumors from obtaining the blood supply needed to fuel their growth. Similarly, in studies of breast cancer cells, garlic and onion phytochemicals caused cell death or halted cell division, which prevents the cancer cells from multiplying.[30]

Onions, garlic, and their family members also contain flavonoids and phenols. White onions aren't as rich in these antioxidant compounds as yellow and red onions, but shallots are especially high in polyphenol levels. Red onions are particularly rich in quercetin and flavonoid antioxidant molecules called anthocyanins (also abundant in berries). Quercetin can contribute to preventing damaged cells from advancing to cancer and also has anti-inflammatory effects that may contribute to cancer prevention.[31]

Onions and the other vegetables of the *Allium* genus can be added to any and every vegetable dish for great flavor and anticancer benefits. Remember: They must be eaten raw and chewed well or chopped finely before cooking to initiate the chemical reaction that forms the protective sulfur compounds.

M: Mushrooms

Mushrooms are valuable in many ways. They are vital in the ecosystem of our planet as a natural recycler, breaking down fallen trees into simpler compounds, for instance. They also help detoxify environments contaminated with wastes that we humans produce. And they are one of the most important human foods on the planet. Both dried and cooked mushrooms add unique flavors and textures to vegetable and bean dishes and soups.

Mushrooms have long been regarded around the world as a gourmet cuisine, but now they are finally being recognized as an essential food for health, with tremendous powers to enhance our immune system function. Recently, a number of antitumor agents have been identified in various mushrooms with numerous mechanisms of action. Mushrooms' specialized lectins (called antigen-binding lectins) can recognize and bind to abnormal cells and cancer cells, labeling the cell for destruction by the immune system, while its compounds also prevent abnormal cells from dividing and replicating.[32] Mushroom phytochemicals also enhance the activity of natural killer cells, that is, specialized immune cells that attack and destroy virus-infected and cancerous cells.[33]

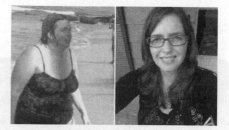

IN THEIR OWN WORDS

Julie's life was a revolving door of doctor's visits and antibiotics. She discovered that more pharmaceuticals aren't the solution to health problems; nutrient-dense eating is.

BEFORE: More than 225 pounds

AFTER: 150 pounds

My journey to health started fourteen months ago. I was lying on the couch with my three-year-old. Both of us were sick—again. He had a double ear infection, and I had sinusitis and pneumonia. I was on my fifth course of antibiotics in four months. I had been suffering with a headache for months at that point, and my migraine medications had stopped working. I had to go to the doctor to get shots for my migraines, and when they didn't work, I had to go to the urgent care clinic to get stronger shots. I was missing work because of headaches. It was awful.

My total cholesterol was just under 200, and the last time I had seen my doctor, he had told me that I needed to start watching my blood pressure because it was high too. My polycystic ovary syndrome was out of control. I was taking 300 milligrams of progesterone, but the pain was still horrible.

I knew I needed to make a change, but I had tried all kinds of diets, with no success. I felt hopeless. One life-changing day, I happened to hear Dr. Fuhrman on television speak about a different kind of food pyramid and a way to nourish my body and lose weight at the same time. I was inspired. I committed to following the nutritarian diet style for six weeks. I figured what did I have to lose? Six weeks later I had lost 22 pounds.

I now weigh 150 pounds. And I haven't had a single migraine headache. My polycystic ovary syndrome has disappeared. I don't even get premenstrual syndrome anymore! I don't get sick like I did before either. My husband says he isn't afraid I'm going to die in my sleep, like he used to be because I snored so much and would stop breathing. I have energy. I can play with my kids. I'm glad to say I'm off all of my medications—progesterone gone! Allegra, gone! Albuterol, gone! Flonase, gone! Sudafed, gone! All migraine medications, gone!

In one recent Chinese study, women who ate at least 10 grams of fresh mushrooms each day (roughly one button mushroom) decreased their risk of breast cancer by 64 percent.[34] Plus, mushrooms contain aromatase inhibitors, compounds that can block the production of estrogen. Even the most commonly eaten mushrooms—white, cremini, and portobello—have high antiaromatase activity.[35]

Mushrooms also contain powerful angiogenesis inhibitors.[36] All types of mushrooms have a wide variety of anticancer properties, and mushroom phytochemicals have shown anticancer effects against stomach, colorectal, and prostate cancers as well.[37] Because angiogenesis is also required for the growth of fat cells, mushrooms oppose fat deposition on the body while simultaneously working against the growth of cancer cells.

Mushrooms have other anti-obesity effects. Their chemical properties oppose insulin, which helps lower blood sugar levels and interferes with fat deposition on the body. Mushrooms are the true weight-loss miracle food.[38] It's fascinating how mushrooms work to induce weight loss and reverse diabetes and lower blood sugar. Since they are so low in calories and satisfying to eat, you would expect that eating them in place of meat, oil, and bread would help you lose weight; but that isn't the only way they help. They also block enzymes that break down carbohydrates into simple sugars, which allows the body to maintain lower sugar surges in the blood when it's breaking down foods that contain carbohydrates.[39]

Mushrooms are even better than probiotics at increasing the diversity of healthy bacteria inside the gut. Mushrooms also foster resistance against pathogenic bacteria such as salmonella and *Clostridium difficile*.[40] Furthermore, they increase salivary and mucosal immunoglobulin A, which further increases resistance to bowel infection and inflammation.[41]

Keep in mind that you should cook most mushrooms before you eat them: The simple white, cremini, and portobello mushrooms contain a potentially carcinogenic substance called agaritine. Cooking them significantly reduces their agaritine content.[42]

B: Berries (and Pomegranates)

Blueberries, raspberries, strawberries, and blackberries are vibrantly colored with antioxidant phytochemicals, and they are some of the highest antioxidant foods in existence. The deep red, blue, and purple pigments of berries are produced by anthocyanins, which are concentrated in the skins of the fruits. Flavonoids are not merely antioxidants; they are thought to have a number of additional beneficial effects in the body that are unrelated to their antioxidant capacity. Several studies have shown that high flavonoid intake is associated with considerable risk reductions (up to 45 percent) for coronary heart disease.[43] The plentiful antioxidant content of berries helps to reduce blood pressure and inflammation, to prevent DNA damage that leads to cancer, to protect the brain against oxidative damage, and to stimulate the body's own antioxidant enzymes.[44]

Ellagic acid, another antioxidant abundant in both berries and pomegranates, was found in the 1980s to block the formation of tumors, providing the initial evidence that these fruits were anti-cancer foods.[45] Antioxidant activity contributes to protection against cancers, since oxidative damage of DNA can cause cancerous changes in cells. The antioxidant phytochemicals in berries and pomegranates also prevent carcinogens from binding DNA and promote DNA repair, which leads to a reduced likelihood of the initiation of cancer.[46]

Berry and pomegranate extracts have slowed cell growth or caused cell death in cells from several different human cancer types.[47] Like mushrooms, pomegranates and many berries also have antiangiogenic properties, inhibiting the blood supply to tumors and thus preventing them from receiving the nutrients they need to grow.[48]

Remember: Angiogenic inhibitors also inhibit
fat storage in the body.

Like mushrooms, pomegranates are also one of the few foods that
contain natural aromatase inhibitors—those substances that inhibit
the production of estrogen, which can reduce breast cancer risk.[49]
Furthermore, one recent exciting study demonstrated the powerful
anticancer effects of berries in patients with precancerous esophageal
lesions. Each patient ate strawberries every day for six months. The
results were amazing: Twenty-nine of the thirty-six study patients experienced a decrease in the histological grade of their lesions. In other
words, the progression toward cancer began to reverse, and the risk of
the lesions becoming cancerous decreased.[50]

Can eating more fruit help you lose weight? Apparently so.
Evidence is accumulating that the anthocyanins and polyphenols
in berries and other fruits actually suppress the generation of new
fatty acids by the liver and promote the degradation or breakdown
of fat stores.[51] Polyphenols, a complex mixture of many plant pigments, oppose and reduce hormones that facilitate fat storage while
restoring the body's normal fat-burning metabolism by altering the
balance and presence of bacteria in the gut. They decrease the bacteria that promote fat storage and increase the bacteria that encourage a slim body.[52] A high consumption of polyphenols leads to an
increase in beneficial bacteria that interfere with the breakdown
of complex carbohydrates into simple sugars, which also facilitates
weight reduction.

A 2011 study investigated berry consumption in relation to the risk
of elevated blood pressure. Just one serving per week decreased the risk
of hypertension by 10 percent.[53] New findings published in 2013 from
the Nurses' Health Study support these results with data in younger
women (age twenty-five to forty-two at the beginning of the study)
who were followed for eighteen years. Having three or more weekly

servings of blueberries or strawberries was linked to a 34 percent reduction in the risk of heart attack.[54]

Berry flavonoids seem to act in several different ways to maintain heart health. In human subjects, for instance, researchers found that berries mitigated oxidative stress and decreased the oxidation of LDL, or "bad cholesterol," which helps prevent the production of atherosclerotic plaque. Berry flavonoids were also found to increase the body's blood antioxidant capacity and in some cases even improved lipid levels, blood pressure, and blood glucose levels.

Similarly, higher anthocyanin and berry intake is associated with reduced C-reactive protein, suggesting that berries may curb inflammation. Additional studies have confirmed that berries have anti-inflammatory properties. Berry phytochemicals also may enhance nitric oxide production in the blood vessels, which helps to properly regulate blood pressure.[55] And berries are the only food documented in studies to prevent dementia in later life.[56]

Even during winter, we can get our daily dose of anthocyanins from frozen berries. Fill your freezer with berries in the summer when you can buy them inexpensively right from the farm. Better yet, put some berry bushes in your yard. Include fresh and frozen berries in your diet as often as possible to enjoy these numerous health benefits. Berries and pomegranates have the highest nutrient-to-calorie ratio of all fruits, and they protect against cancer, heart disease, hypertension, diabetes, and dementia.

S: Seeds

Seeds aren't for the birds. They are a lifespan-promoting food for us humans as well, with dramatic anticancer effects. Seeds are nature's way of perpetuating the plant life of planet earth, and they have a stellar scientific record of protecting our health and prolonging our lives in the process. Not only do seeds add their own spectrum of unique disease-fighting substances to the dietary landscape, but the fat in seeds increases the absorption of protective nutrients in vegetables eaten at the same meal. They contain minerals, antioxidants, and micronutrients, including plant sterols, which help to reduce cholesterol. Several seeds and nuts—such as flaxseeds, hemp seeds, chia seeds, and walnuts—are rich in omega-3 fatty acids, which are beneficial for heart and brain health.[57] Seeds and nuts act like a fat sponge in the digestive tract, preventing all their fat calories from being absorbed.[58] But the real story is that these fat magnets pull out the unhealthy fats from the bloodstream, increasing the cholesterol content of the stool, carrying the bad fats out of the body, and allowing the healthy fats to stay in.

Flax, chia, and sesame seeds are rich in lignans, plant phytoestrogens that protect against cancer. In one study, women who had breast cancer ate muffins that contained flaxseeds; a control group ate muffins without the flax. Within five weeks, the group eating the flaxseed muffins showed a decreased growth of tumor cells, and their previously existing tumor cells were killed off in greater numbers.[59]

Even more surprising was the study of breast cancer patients who consumed a daily average of about 0.3 milligrams of lignans from seeds. The study followed these women for ten years and found a whopping 71 percent lower breast cancer deaths compared with women eating few or no lignans in their diet.[60] This study was powerful for two reasons. First, the mean lignan intake in the largest quartile was so small. One teaspoon of flaxseeds results in 7 milligrams of lignans, and the top dietary lignan group averaged only about one-third of a milligram of lignan daily. This means that a higher seed intake would most likely offer even more protection. Second, the anticancer effects of foods are more powerful before you have cancer and become less effective as cancer progresses, and this study still showed about 70 percent effectiveness from this one factor in women who already had cancer. Remember, this benefit occurred just from this one variable—dietary lignan intake—and didn't include the other anticancer effects of the other G-BOMBS.

Furthermore, hemp seeds, chia seeds, flaxseeds, and walnuts are also rich in the omega-3 fatty acid ALA. Most nuts are richer in linoleic acid, an omega-6 fatty acid. Since omega-3 fats are harder to come by, it's important to eat some foods that are naturally rich in ALA. Research indicates that the regular consumption of ALA reduces the risk of cardiovascular disease and cancer.[61] It is also interesting that some studies indicate that a deficiency in this fatty acid can lead to increased depression and anxiety and a poor ability to cope with stress.[62]

TABLE 7. SUPER SEEDS TO INCLUDE IN YOUR DIET CONTAIN OMEGA-3 ALA AND LIGNANS

SEED	OMEGA-3 ALA (g/oz)	LIGNANS (mg/oz)	% FAT AS OMEGA-3
Chia	4.99	31.92	57.96
Flax	6.39	85.5	54.15
Hemp	2.26	Unknown	17.38
Sesame	0.105	11.2	0.75

Notes: USDA, Agricultural Research Service. National nutrient database for standard reference. http://ndb.nal.usda.gov/ndb/search/list. Higdon J, Drake VJ. Lignans. In: An Evidence-Based Approach to Dietary Phytochemicals. New York: Thieme; 2006:155–161. Nemes SM, Orstat V. Evaluation of a microwave-assisted extraction method for lignan quantification in flaxseed cultivars and selected oil seeds. Food Anal Methods. 2012;5:551–563.

Build a strong nutritional foundation by eating G-BOMBS every day.

By eating significant portions of G-BOMBS, we consistently flood our bodies with their spectrum of phytochemicals that work synergistically to boost immune function and prevent cancer from developing. There is an additional perk too: These same foods protect against heart disease, diabetes, and other devastating chronic illnesses that commonly plague modern Americans.

As you begin to increase your intake of high-nutrient food and reduce your exposure to unhealthful processed foods such as sugar, salt, and oils, you'll start to enjoy, more and more, healthful foods. Over time, your taste preferences will adapt as you make healthy choices, and you'll start to appreciate more subtle flavors. It works. Eat healthfully, and over time you'll *prefer* eating healthfully.

Don't Forget the Tomato Sauce

This discussion of the amazing power of modern nutritional science wouldn't be complete without considering carotenoids and tomatoes. The levels of carotenoids in your body's tissues are a good indicator of your overall health because those levels parallel the levels of plant-derived phytochemicals in general. In a study of more than thirteen thousand American adults, low blood levels of carotenoids were found to be an accurate predictor of earlier death. Lower levels of total carotenoids, alpha-carotene, and lycopene in the blood were linked to increased risk of death from all causes; of all the carotenoids, very low blood lycopene was the strongest predictor of mortality.[63]

Lycopene is the signature carotenoid in tomatoes. In fact, 85 percent of the lycopene Americans consume comes from tomatoes.[64] (Other foods rich in lycopene include red peppers, beets, cherries, and papaya; see Table 8 on page 122.) Lycopene is perhaps best known for its anticancer properties. It also concentrates in the male reproductive system, which makes it an effective protection against prostate cancer.[65]

Ingested phytochemicals have been shown in animal studies to absorb ultraviolet radiation and protect against sun damage. Green tea catechins and flavonols found in apples, cinnamon, berries, and beans have already demonstrated benefits. Researchers recently found that the consumption of tomato paste reduced skin damage from ultraviolet radiation *and* curtailed concomitant DNA damage, which simultane-ously limited the risk of sun-related skin aging *and* cancer.[66]

Lycopene also works wonders for the heart and blood vessels. Many observational studies have noted the connection between high levels of blood lycopene and a lower risk of heart attack. For example, a study in men found that low serum lycopene was associated with increased plaque in the carotid artery and tripled the risk of cardio-vascular events compared with higher levels.[67] In a study that exam-ined women in four different quartiles according to blood lycopene levels, researchers observed that the women in the top three quartiles were 50 percent less likely to have cardiovascular disease than the lowest quartile.[68]

Similarly, a 2004 analysis of the Physicians' Health Study data found a 39 percent decrease in stroke risk in men with the highest blood levels of lycopene.[69] For twelve years, physicians in Finland fol-lowed one thousand men, regularly testing their blood carotenoid levels. Men with the highest lycopene levels were 55 percent less likely to suffer a stroke than men with the lowest lycopene levels.[70] Previous data from this same group showed that higher lycopene levels often lowered the risk of heart attack.[71]

Lycopene is also an extremely potent antioxidant. According to several studies, the increase of tomato products in the diet helped guard against LDL oxidation, an early step in the formation of ath-erosclerotic plaque.[72] Another study found that a tomato-rich diet im-proved the body's endothelial function, that is, its ability to regulate blood pressure within the inner lining of blood vessels. Oxidation impairs endothelial function.[73] And this result occurred after only two weeks!

Lycopene may also protect against cardiovascular disease. Early ev-idence seems to indicate that lycopene inhibits HMG-CoA reductase, the enzyme responsible for producing cholesterol and the one targeted by cholesterol-lowering statin drugs. Numerous trials have shown that by adding extra tomato products to their diets, subjects reduced their blood cholesterol levels. A meta-analysis of twelve trials found that daily supplemental tomato products—approximately 1 cup of tomato juice or 3 to 4 tablespoons of tomato paste per day— reduced LDL cholesterol by 10 percent. This is comparable to the results obtained with low doses of statin drugs—minus the nasty side effects, of course.[74]

Lycopene also has anti-inflammatory effects and may prevent the excessive proliferation of vascular smooth muscle cells, a contributor to atherosclerotic plaque.[75]

TABLE 8. LYCOPENE CONTENT OF SOME FOODS

FOOD	LYCOPENE CONTENT (mcg)
Tomato sauce (1 cup)	41,875
Tomato paste (½ cup)	18,843
Watermelon (1 cup)	6,979
Tomatoes (raw, 1 cup)	4,632
Grapefruit (pink, 1 fruit)	3,490
Guava (1 fruit)	2,862
Papaya (1 cup)	2,559

Of course, lycopene isn't the only nutrient in tomatoes. They are also rich in other carotenoids; numerous vitamins, such as vitamins C and E; and flavonol antioxidants. While lycopene is likely the carotenoid with the most potent antioxidant, a combination of carotenoids is even more effective than any single one; they work synergistically to provide the greatest health benefit. Their full interaction triggers good health. A single pill or individual supplement can't compete. In a given year, a typical American will eat about 92 pounds of tomatoes.[76] Enjoy those 92 pounds!—and continue to add more. Add fresh tomatoes to every salad. Mix some diced or unsulfured sun-dried tomatoes into your next bowl of soup. Enjoy homemade tomato sauces and soups. But watch out for the sodium content of ketchup and many other tomato products; low-sodium or no-salt alternatives are the best. And because carotenoids are best absorbed when accompanied by healthy fats, make sure to add them to a salad that includes seeds or has a nut-based dressing.[77] Lycopene is also more absorbable when tomatoes are cooked, so enjoy a variety of raw and cooked tomatoes in your daily diet.[78]

CHAPTER FIVE

Nutritarian
Boot Camp

A nutritarian diet style is more than just a way to eat—it's an attitude, a mind-set, a method that you can follow for a lifetime. As you begin your journey as a nutritarian you'll start to take control of your own health and life. When you focus on eating the healthiest foods possible, you eat to live better, without the fear of disease and death, which makes for a more peaceful and pleasurable life.

The foundation of this program are foods that ensure that your body is supplied with everything it needs for optimal health. This nutritarian diet style enables you to lose weight and keep it off permanently, without experiencing hunger or depriving yourself of food. It is the healthiest and most effective eating style in the world. You'll never want or need to diet ever again.

My dietary advice is based on eating large quantities of nutrient-rich foods and fewer foods with minimal nutritional value.

A low-calorie, high-nutrient diet slows down the aging process, helps repair cells, reduces inflammation, and helps rid the body of toxins. High-nutrient, low-calorie foods contain a great deal of fiber and take up a lot of room in the stomach. As you consume a smaller number of calories, you simultaneously eat a larger quantity of food, which satiates your hunger and blunts your appetite. Meeting the body's micronutrient needs also helps suppress food cravings—finally putting an end to that vicious cycle of addiction, toxic hunger, and overeating. The more nutrient-dense food you consume, the more you will be satisfied with fewer calories, and the less you will crave fat and high-calorie foods. Once you begin to learn which foods make the grade by having a high proportion of nutrients to calories, you're on your way to lifelong weight control and improved health. Though it is easy to understand that colorful plants are nutrient-rich, and processed foods and animal products lack a significant load of antioxidants and phytochemicals, it is helpful for many people to see actual scores of the nutrients contained in various foods. Every food or diet can be evaluated using this formula, and this visual tool can help motivate you to eat more high-nutrient vegetation and less processed foods and animal products.

The ANDI Scoring System

To help visualize the H = N / C equation and make it practical, I created the *aggregate nutrient density index,* or ANDI. It is presently used at Whole Foods Market grocery stores to illustrate which natural foods have the highest nutrient-per-calorie density. The ANDI ranks the nutrient density of many common foods on the basis of how many nutrients they deliver to your body for each calorie consumed. It also helps you visualize how nutrient dense green vegetables are and how foods compare with one another in nutrient density. I set the highest ANDI score at 1,000.

Food labels list only a few nutrients, but ANDIs are based on twenty-eight important nutritional parameters. The ANDI is a simple way to help you identify and eat larger amounts of nutrient-rich foods. The higher the ANDI and the greater percentage of those foods in your diet, the better your health will be. Table 9 shows some ANDI scores. How do the foods you eat rate?

TABLE 9. ANDI SCORES

FOOD	SCORE	FOOD	SCORE
Collard greens	1,000	Cabbage	434
Kale	1,000	Broccoli	340
Mustard greens	1,000	Cauliflower	315
Watercress	1,000	Bell peppers	265
Swiss chard	895	Mushrooms	238
Bok choy	865	Asparagus	205
Spinach	707	Tomatoes	186
Arugula	604	Strawberries	182
Romaine lettuce	510	Sweet potatoes	181
Brussels sprouts	490	Zucchini	164
Carrots	458	Artichokes	145

FOOD	SCORE	FOOD	SCORE
Blueberries	132	Eggs	34
Iceberg lettuce	127	Salmon	34
Grapes	119	Milk (1 percent)	31
Pomegranates	119	Bananas	30
Cantaloupes	118	Walnuts	30
Onions	109	Whole wheat bread	30
Flaxseeds	103	Almonds	28
Edamame	98	Avocados	28
Oranges	98	Brown rice	28
Cucumbers	87	Plain yogurt (low fat)	28
Tofu	82	White potatoes	28
Sesame seeds	74	Cashews	27
Lentils	72	Oatmeal	26
Peaches	65	Chicken breasts	24
Green peas	64	Ground beef (85 percent lean)	21
Kidney beans	64	Feta cheese	20
Sunflower seeds	64	French fries	12
Cherries	55	Apple juice	11
Pineapples	54	Cheddar cheese	11
Apples	53	White pasta (unfortified)	11
Mangoes	53	Olive oil	10
Peanut butter	51	White bread (unfortified)	9
Corn	45	Vanilla ice cream	9
Pistachio nuts	37	Corn chips	7
Shrimp	36	Cola	1

Note: The following nutrients were included: fiber, calcium, iron, magnesium, phosphorus, potassium, zinc, copper, manganese, selenium, vitamin A, beta carotene, alpha carotene, lycopene, lutein and zeaxanthin, vitamin E, vitamin C, thiamin, riboflavin, niacin, pantothenic acid, vitamin B6, folate, vitamin B12, choline, vitamin K, phytosterols, glucosinolates, angiogenesis inhibitors, organosulfides, aromatase inhibitors, resistant starch, resveratrol plus ORAC score. ORAC (Oxygen Radical Absorbance Capacity) is a measure of the antioxidant or radical scavenging capacity of a food.

Getting generous amounts of micronutrients per calorie with unprocessed, natural food is the goal of the nutritarian diet style. This
way, your body is nourished with a comprehensive array of both discovered and undiscovered nutrients in their natural states—just as
nature intended. The ANDI is a tool to help you visualize the value of
eating more greens and other colorful plant foods and less processed
foods and animal products. It's not the only thing to consider for superior health, however. Remember that weight loss and longevity are
both the products of a wide array of nutrients, not just a select few
healthful foods. You have to eat a broad variety of nutrient-rich, natural foods: green vegetables, various fruits, beans, seeds, and nuts, for instance, as well as cooked mushrooms and raw onions—the G-BOMBS
explored in the last chapter.

The ANDI also helps you understand that the standard American
diet is dramatically and dangerously nutrient deficient and fails to provide hundreds of important plant-derived, immunity-building compounds. As the diagram below shows, almost 55 percent of the calories
Americans consume come from processed foods, which contain hardly
any micronutrients.[1] The ANDI makes it easy to compare the micronutrient load of carrots, tomatoes, and broccoli, the foods Americans
eat very little of, with that of white pasta, French fries, and apple juice,
foods Americans eat lots of.

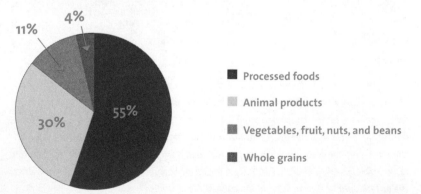

At the same time, we aren't eating enough fruits, beans, seeds and nuts, and vegetables, which leaves us lacking in the most essential health-promoting compounds. To make matters worse, white potatoes and ketchup make up almost half of the 10 percent of the unrefined plant foods that American eat, so clearly Americans eat an insignificant amount of natural plant foods. My clinical experience and research findings demonstrate that low-nutrient eating drives overeating behavior and food cravings. A properly nourished body, however, will be satisfied with the right number of calories, will be resistant to putting on visceral (internal) body fat, and will naturally gravitate toward its ideal weight.

It's not enough to eat foods rich in phytochemicals, antioxidants, vitamins, and minerals. We also have to avoid foods that are toxic or drive up dangerous hormones such as insulin and IGF-1 to dangerously high levels.

Glucose, Insulin, and Good and Bad Carbs

Human cells need energy to function. And the body's primary source of energy is *glucose,* a simple sugar that comes from the body digesting foods that contain carbohydrates—basically any food that contains sugar and/or starches. Insulin, a hormone produced by beta cells in your pancreas, allows glucose to move from your bloodstream directly into your body's cells, which provides them with energy.

Under normal conditions, glucose rises gradually in the bloodstream as we eat, and the insulin-producing cells in the pancreas monitor that rise. These cells then secrete the appropriate amount of insulin to drive the glucose into the body's tissues, lowering the level in the bloodstream to an appropriate range. High levels of glucose cause your pancreas to produce high levels of insulin to flush glucose out of your bloodstream and into your body's cells, where it can safely be converted into energy or, if not needed for energy, stored as fat. Diabetes is essentially the presence of high levels of glucose in your bloodstream.

A high amount of insulin, however, is also harmful because excess insulin supports and drives fat storage (*lipogenesis*), while simultaneously suppressing fat removal (*lipolysis*). Increased levels of insulin also promote angiogenesis, that is, the growth of new blood vessels that feed fat cells and ultimately enable a larger body mass. Stored body fat acts like a barrier to insulin function, so the pancreas responds by producing more and more insulin.

Foods with high levels of glucose, then, force your pancreas to overproduce insulin, which can lead to obesity, type 2 diabetes, and specific types of cancer. You can measure these glucose levels through glycemic index (GI), which evaluates the blood glucose response per gram of carbohydrate in particular foods. It works on a scale of 1 to 100, with 1 being the best. GI measures how high blood sugar levels typically rise after you eat a particular food. Glycemic load (GL) supplies a similar ranking but is thought to be more meaningful because it takes into account the blood sugar response to a common portion size of each food rather than a fixed number of grams.

Carbohydrates, the source of glucose, can be categorized as unrefined or refined—good or bad carbs, respectively. Refined, or processed, carbohydrates have been stripped of their fiber and nutrients, both of which slow down the absorption of sugar. Their absence, in turn, results in high GI and GL values, much higher than values in unrefined carbohydrates.

Foods with a high GL include sugar, white bread, and sweetened breakfast cereals; low-GL foods include beans, intact whole grains, fresh fruits, and vegetables (see Table 10, on page 133). White potatoes, although they are a whole plant food, are also high in GI and GL, and this is the reason why potato consumption of even one serving a day is associated with an increased risk of type 2 diabetes.[2]

Foods with high GI and GL values produce spikes in blood glucose levels, which lead to heightened secretion of insulin by the pancreas. Large quantities of high-GL foods increase the risk of diabetes and several cancers, especially colorectal cancer.[3] For example, the high GL of white potato is responsible for its link to a higher incidence of colorectal cancer.[4] This is further supported by the fact that the diabetes- and colon cancer–promoting potential in white potato is noted predominantly in people who are overweight and therefore have a heightened insulin response to GL. In addition, researchers were careful to separate the effects of both unhealthy toppings used on potatoes and their method of preparation. They showed that as the insulin resistance of the subjects increased, the negative effects of white potato became more pronounced. This means that high-glycemic, insulin-promoting foods are more cancer-causing in overweight people compared with thin, active individuals without insulin resistance.

Consuming foods with a high GL increases heart disease risk as well. One study followed subjects in Italy for eight years. Subjects were divided into four groups according to their intake of high-GI and high-GL foods, and the incidence of coronary heart disease was recorded. In women, the groups with the greatest intake of high-GI foods had a 68 percent greater risk of heart disease than those with the lowest intake. Analyzing by GL revealed an even more pronounced effect: Women with the highest intake of high-GL foods were more than twice as likely to develop heart disease compared with women with the lowest intake.[5] A similar study performed in men found an increased risk of heart attack in men who ate the greatest quantities of high-GI and high-GL foods.[6]

Refined carbohydrates aren't the only macronutrients that raise insulin levels. High-protein foods like meat do, too. Certain foods cause an insulin response over and above what would be reflected by their GL. This effect is reflected in a food's insulin index. When you mix animal products and oils with sugar or white flour, your body's insulin response spikes even more dramatically.[7] A plate of fried chicken and biscuits, for example, would be more hormonally dangerous than biscuits alone.

In Their Own Words

Catherine discovered that weight loss isn't the only benefit to incorporating superior nutrition into her life. She also found that food is "healing medicine" that provides "life-giving energy" for her body.

BEFORE: 166 pounds

AFTER: 128 pounds

Last summer I knew I had to do something about my weight. My fiftieth birthday was looming, and I couldn't bear the thought of reaching this milestone with an extra 30 to 40 pounds on my body. I also wanted to feel better. More often than not, my mediocre eating habits had left me feeling chaotic, lethargic, and overwhelmed, in addition to having a "meno-pot" belly and fat rolls on my back and hips! I have struggled with anxiety and attention deficit issues all of my life, and my standard American diet provided me with little ammunition for effective coping and flourishing.

I had been looking for a guide to healthy eating that wasn't complicated, and I struck gold when I discovered Dr. Fuhrman's website, which enabled me to carefully track my nutritarian journey.

I was uncertain at first as I roamed grocery store aisles buying kale, collard greens, and leeks; sunflower seeds, walnuts and cashews, currants, Medjool dates and pomegranates, and mushrooms of all kinds. Yet within a matter of days, I was more alert and energetic—the brain "fog" or "malaise" that had hovered over my life for so long seemed to have lifted.

When I first committed to healthy eating at the end of August, I weighed 166 pounds. My original plan had been to follow Dr. Fuhrman's nutritarian diet until my fiftieth birthday in late November. But I soon realized that I was on a life-changing and lifelong journey in which food was about healing and wholeness. I'm struck by how little I knew about nutrition. I knew about the benefits of exercise, but I didn't know much about how food could be such healing medicine and life-giving energy for my body. I love that I'm eating to protect my body against cancer and dementia and helping ensure that I can live a healthy, full life into old age.

TABLE 10. GLYCEMIC LOAD PER CUP OF COMMON HIGH-CARBOHYDRATE FOODS

FOOD	GLYCEMIC LOAD	FOOD	GLYCEMIC LOAD
Cauliflower	Negligible	Barley	13
Strawberries	1	Navy beans	13
Cashews	2	Rolled/steel-cut oats	13
Oranges	4	Black-eyed peas	14
Split peas	4	Quinoa	16
Black beans	6	Corn	18
Watermelon	6	Sweet potatoes	19
Red kidney beans	7	White bread (2 slices)	20
Butternut squash	8	White pasta	21
Green peas	8	Brown rice	24
Kiwis	8	Millet	26
Apples	9	White potatoes	29
Beets	9	White rice	29
Lentils	9	Cola (12 oz can)	32
Whole wheat	11		

Notes: Atkinson FS, Foster-Powell K, Brand-Miller JC. International tables of glycemic index and glycemic load values: 2008. Diabetes Care. 2008;31(12):2281–2283. Foster-Powell K, Holt SH, Brand-Miller JC. International table of glycemic index and glycemic load values: 2002. Am J Clin Nutr. 2002;76(1):5–56.

Except for white potatoes, natural whole plant foods do *not* have a very high GL. For the most part, natural foods do not create a heightened glucose and insulin response, though I do advise the overweight or diabetic to avoid white potatoes. And if you're significantly overweight or diabetic, I also recommend limiting brown rice, millet, and even sweet potatoes, as high-GL foods are generally considered 20 and above. It's interesting that today's fast-growing, large "Irish" russet and Idaho potatoes aren't at all like the many varieties of small, multicolored wild potatoes that originated in the Andes Mountains. These contained more than ten times the phytonutrients and were much higher in fiber and resistant starch than the russets and Idahos. Which means they had a lower GL than modern-day, overly bred potatoes.

It's not the quantity of carbohydrates that's necessarily bad. It's the *quality* of the carbohydrate that can make it so bad for you. Low-quality carbohydrates, which are generally refined and highly glycemic, are calorically dense and lack sufficient protective antioxidants. Such processed foods are addictive and promote fat storage over and above their caloric load because of their hormone-promoting effects. A diet heavy in low-quality carbohydrates is largely responsible for our overweight and metabolically challenged population.

High-quality carbohydrates, on the other hand, are nutritionally valuable and contain predominantly slowly digestible and resistant starches that limit their GL. Foods such as green peas and red beans, though packed with carbohydrates, are slowly digested and do not spike glucose in the bloodstream. These high-quality carbohydrates are not only health-promoting, but they also promote a favorable body weight and slim waist. The combination of their slower glucose absorption with the fibers and nutrients they contain prevents the body from storing fat, whereas white bread, soda, and French fries, with the same caloric load, are quickly digested and highly obesogenic, or obesity-causing. Other favorable high-carbohydrate foods include cauliflower, chickpeas, English peas, split peas, various squashes, turnips, and rutabagas. Of course, raw vegetables, including raw carrots and raw shredded beets, are nutrient-rich, low-glycemic, healthful food choices as well.

Beans, however, head the list of preferred carbohydrate-rich foods. Beans have a low GL and are also high in micronutrients and fiber. I rank beans among the world's most perfect foods. They stabilize blood sugar, blunt your desire for sweets, and help you feel full. Beans contain both insoluble fiber and soluble fiber and are very high in resistant starch—more than any other high-carbohydrate food. Though technically a starch, resistant starch acts more like a fiber by "resisting digestion." Since resistant starch passes through the small intestine undigested, a significant number of the calories derived from a bean's carbohydrate load is not fully absorbed.

So consider beans your preferred high-carbohydrate food. Among your more common choices (and there are lots of uncommon varieties as well) are chickpeas, black-eyed peas, black beans, split peas, lima beans, pinto beans, lentils, red kidney beans, soybeans, cannellini beans, and white beans. You can almost never go wrong with beans.

More Than Calories

Not only does counting calories and eating less not work for long-term weight loss, but it isn't supported by advances in nutritional science or clinical evidence. A nutritionally unsound low-calorie diet is doomed to fail because it increases your cravings and hunger signals. With so few nutrients for your brain, you become more emotional and less able to handle stress. Which means you're more likely to binge on junk food.

Some people have proposed focusing on the caloric density of foods. This, too, is unsustainable, largely because it's too narrow a criterion for evaluating relative food value. Caloric density alone doesn't consider a food's protective anticancer potential or other health benefits. Nor does it account for the *quality* of its carbohydrate content, which includes its fiber content and the proportion of slowly digestible, resistant starch. A diet style with a favorable caloric density needs to consider micronutrient density and overall health benefits. A diet with a high amount of micronutrients per calorie, and with a low hormonal index (meaning insulin and IGF-1), is more descriptive of what is healthful. Such a diet also has a favorable low caloric density overall.

At the same time, if you overemphasize calorie density, you might be encouraged to exclude from your diet seeds and nuts, which have a high caloric density. Nuts and seeds have a very high count of calories per gram, almost five times higher than that of meat, yet as discussed in the last chapter, they have been shown to promote weight loss and dramatically enhance health and longevity. Meat has the opposite effect.[8] It may promote general cell growth, but it also stimulates fat storage hormones. Plus, when your diet contains more nuts and seeds instead of foods high in refined carbohydrates or animal products, the disease-promoting and cancer-promoting hormones insulin and IGF-1 are reduced. Substituting seeds and nuts, calorie for calorie, for carbohydrates or animal products results in lower body fat storage, which makes it easier for you to maintain a favorable weight. This makes the emphasis on calorie density in opposition to the preponderance of scientific evidence.

It is common in the diet industry to structure a new diet book or plan around one factor that makes a diet look favorable and inflate the importance of that factor, while almost ignoring all the other factors that are important. For example, besides caloric density being too narrow a criteria to structure a diet plan around, the low-glycemic diet, the alkaline diet, the high-fiber diet, the low-sugar diet, the high-starch diet, the low-fat diet, and many more are also simply incorrect in their emphasis and simplicity. When you give up on diet plans, you recognize that eating healthfully cannot be summed up with a narrow focus—it must be comprehensively inclusive of all healthful parameters.

Lower Levels of IGF-I Lead to a Longer Life

IGF-1 is one of the body's most important growth promoters during fetal and childhood development. Later in life, however, it accelerates the aging process and promotes the growth and replication of cells, which often leads to cancer.

An elevated IGF-1 level is linked to an increased risk of all major cancers, including cancers of the colon, breast, and prostate.[9] It stimulates mitosis (cell division) and inhibits apoptosis (a process leading to cell death). This means that IGF-1 not only promotes the spread of cancerous cells, it also inhibits the immune system's ability to identify and kill abnormal cells before they become cancerous (apoptosis). Furthermore, as we age, high circulating IGF-1 levels promote the replication of injured cells that otherwise would not become malignant.

Heightened IGF-1 levels also promote the growth and proliferation of tumor cells and enhance tumor cell survival, adhesion, migration, invasion, angiogenesis, and metastatic growth.[10] Reduced IGF-1 levels in adulthood are also associated with reduced oxidative stress, decreased inflammation, enhanced insulin sensitivity, and longer lifespan.[11]

But the big story here is IGF-1 and cancer. So many dieters have jumped on the high-protein bandwagon, eating egg whites, fish, and lean meats under the false assumption that they're eating healthfully. In truth, however, this kind of diet is fueling an explosion of cancer. The nutritarian diet is specifically designed to maximize cancer-protective nutrients from foods and minimize or negate cancer-promoting dietary practices.

Unquestionably, IGF-1 is a major player in the causation of breast and prostate cancer. The European Prospective Investigation into Cancer and Nutrition (EPIC) found that elevated IGF-1 levels were associated with a 40 percent increased risk of developing breast cancer for women older than fifty.[12] In the Nurses' Health Study, high IGF-1 levels were associated with a doubled risk of breast cancer in premenopausal women.[13] Additional human studies, reviews of the literature, and five meta-analyses have also found an association between elevated IGF-1 levels and the development of breast cancer.[14] The most recent of these showed a strong correlation with the most common estrogen-positive breast cancers in both premenopausal and postmenopausal women.

Higher levels of IGF-1 were observed in overweight women, consumers of alcohol, and those who ate a diet higher in animal products.

In other words, higher IGF-1 levels promote common cancers. End of controversy. Not only that, but excess IGF-1 also promotes dementia in humans, while lower IGF-1 levels enhance brain function in later years. Elevated circulating IGF-1 levels have been found in patients with Alzheimer's disease, and reduced IGF-1 signaling reduces symptoms of neurodegeneration.[15] In muscle tissues that require IGF-1 for proper functioning or repair in adulthood, local production of IGF-1 from muscular exertion compensates for the lower circulating IGF-1 levels. So lower levels are longevity-promoting and have no apparent drawbacks.

Which Foods Raise IGF-1 Levels?

Since the principle dietary factor that determines IGF-1 levels is animal protein, the excessive meat, fowl, seafood, and dairy intake common in our society is responsible for high circulating IGF-1 levels. When many of us were children, we were taught that animal products were good for us because they were a biologically complete protein that was essential for good health. Research in the past ten years, however, has shown conclusively that high biological protein is the most damaging feature of animal products.[16]

Milk products raise IGF-1 levels the most, though this is most likely the result of other bioactive growth-promoting compounds in addition to their high protein content. Ten different observational studies and several interventional studies have confirmed a positive correlation between milk and heightened levels of IGF-1.[17] Take prostate cancer for instance, which seems to be particularly sensitive to IGF-1 levels. The risk of developing this cancer increases in direct proportion to an increased consumption of dairy and meat.[18] Researchers tracked more than twenty-one thousand men in the Physicians' Health Study for twenty-eight years and found that those who had one serving of milk a day had double the risk of dying from prostate cancer compared with men who rarely drank milk.[19] Meat consumption was also shown to raise IGF-1 levels in this study. Several other studies have confirmed that meat, poultry, and fish raise IGF-1 levels.[20]

"Free IGF-1," rather than the IGF-1 that is bound to proteins, has the growth-promoting biological activity that promotes cancer; so if the IGF-1 binding proteins are reduced, more free IGF-1 is available to perform its nefarious duties. Therefore, it is important to note, the higher consumption of saturated fat from meat and cheese in conjunction with the high level of animal protein makes things worse by decreasing levels of the IGF-1 binding proteins, thus increasing free IGF-1 levels in the circulation.

But it's not only animal products that raise IGF-1 levels. Refined carbohydrates do too, because they cause rapid increases in insulin levels, which lead to an increase in IGF-1 signaling, a major factor in the connection between diabetes and cancer.[21] And heightened levels of insulin raise IGF-1, which is another reason why a high-glycemic diet promotes cancer. At the same time, by adhering to a cell's insulin receptor, IGF-1 can also act like insulin to promote fat storage. When both are elevated, you have a cancer-promoting sandwich—like a ham and cheese sandwich on white bread. Regularly consuming high-glycemic foods with animal protein, a common staple of the SAD, promotes cancer. Everyday dishes like pizza, spaghetti and meatballs, a hamburger on a bun, fish and chips, and steak and fries are responsible for promoting a cancer epidemic in this country.

Isolated soy protein, found in protein powders and meat substitutes, may also be problematic because the protein is unnaturally concentrated and its amino acid profile is very similar to that of animal protein. Dietary interventions using isolated soy protein confirmed that it raised IGF-1 levels more than soybeans.[22] Such excessive IGF-1–promoting effects were not seen with tofu or unprocessed soybeans alone.[23] A variety of beans in the diet is most healthful, rather than an excessive dependence on just soy foods, especially processed soy foods, as they may raise IGF-1 levels too much.

If you want to live to be one hundred years old, the road to getting there is clear. Centenarians have low levels of IGF-1 and high levels of anti-inflammatory molecules from nutrient-dense plant foods. A diet high in phytochemicals, resulting in lower levels of oxidative stress, coupled with a reduction in IGF-1 is the secret to longevity and protection against cancer.[24]

The amount of animal products that can safely be added to a diet is not clearly defined; however, averaging more than 1 ounce a day for women and 1.5 ounces a day for men is likely risky. The IGF-1 curve starts to increase considerably above these levels.[25] Since this is an area of evolving science, this is just an estimated guideline based on the information available today.

When I wrote *Fasting and Eating for Health* in 1995, I noted that the only scientifically documented way to slow aging and prolong life was through restricting calories in a nutritional environment of micronutrient adequacy. The advancements in science over the past twenty years have shown that protein restriction is even more lifespan-promoting than episodic calorie restriction, and the benefits of calorie restriction can be negated if the intake of animal protein is too high—potentially even at levels just above 10 percent of total dietary calories.

Restricting calories and reducing IGF-1 signaling are the only two well-established means of increasing lifespan. Both are characterized by slimness and decreased insulin levels; however, most scientists in this field believe that the mechanism that extends lifespan so dramatically is the effect that calorie restriction has on keeping IGF-1 levels low.

The pivotal investigation that changed the playing field was a six-year study published in 2008 with members of the Calorie Restriction Society. Unlike the lower IGF-1 levels seen in calorie-restricted animals, the study found that the IGF-1 levels in calorie-restricted humans were *not* significantly different from those of a control group eating the SAD.[26] Scientists were surprised and first thought that caloric restriction does not extend human life like it does in animals. The researchers then noted that the study group eating fewer calories was consuming more animal protein as a percentage of total calories than the SAD. Apparently, the animal protein was inhibiting the drop in IGF-1 they had expected.

When they compared those unfavorable IGF-1 levels in the study participants with the IGF-1 levels found in vegans, they saw dramatically lowered IGF-1 levels in the vegans even though the vegans weren't restricting calories. This explained the lack of the expected benefits in the calorie-restricted subjects. Further investigations continued in this field, eventually quantifying the differences in IGF-1 levels and the IGF-1–raising potential for various diet styles and foods utilizing forty-seven hundred participants, further confirming that animal protein intake was primarily responsible for maintaining the elevations in IGF-1 levels.[27]

Restricting calories and maintaining a favorable body weight, in an environment of adequate micronutrient intake, dramatically increases longevity and reduces cancer risk in humans, but only if the animal protein intake is significantly restricted. Furthermore, reducing animal protein intake is more powerful at enhancing lifespan than chronic calorie restriction in humans.

Exercise can also lower IGF-1 levels. A study published in the *American Journal of Clinical Nutrition* investigated the effects of long-distance running and diet on reducing IGF-1, comparing levels in vegans and SAD eaters, both of whom were relatively sedentary.[28] They contacted local running clubs to study runners averaging 48 miles a week, and local vegetarian societies to find healthy-eating vegans. The results were impressive:

	AVERAGE BMI	AVERAGE IGF-1
Vegans	21.3	139
Runners	21.6	177
SAD eaters	26.5	201

The study noted that the low-protein-consuming vegans were not eating a low-fat diet. They were eating plenty of nuts and seeds and even used olive oil. In all groups, plasma IGF-1 levels correlated linearly with dietary protein intake, and reduced animal protein intake had a more powerful effect at reducing levels of IGF-1 and inflammatory markers compared with endurance exercise.

The average daily protein intake in the vegans was 0.73 grams per kilogram of body weight, whereas the other groups consumed about twice that amount. Also of interest was that IGF-1 was the major difference, not testosterone and other sex hormones, which did not differ significantly between the groups.

Red Meat, Gut Bacteria, and Heart Disease

The high-protein intake from animal products doesn't just accelerate aging and produce cancer. Excessive meat intake has also been associated with an elevated risk of cardiovascular death.[29] For example, combined data from the Nurses' Health Study and Health Professionals Follow-up Study, which together examined more than 120,000 people, estimated that each serving of red meat a day raises the risk of cardiovascular death by a whopping 18 percent.

In Their Own Words

Claudia was a "Vegjunkatarian," mistaking her avoidance of meat for healthy eating until she turned to a nutritarian approach and realized true health with renewed energy.

BEFORE: 120 pounds

AFTER: 90 pounds

I've been a vegetarian since I was fifteen years old. My vegetarian diet was similar to the disease-promoting diet that most Americans eat, minus the meat, of course. I was addicted to junk foods like pizza, French fries, grilled cheese sandwiches, and vanilla ice cream with chocolate syrup. I seemed to always struggle either to lose weight or keep it off. Eventually I eliminated all dairy products, which brought my cholesterol down to a healthy level, but I was still eating disease-promoting foods.

I was always a low-energy person and didn't like to exercise. Deprivation dieting and exercise were both burdens to me, so I didn't stick with either of them. I also developed a large fibroid on my uterus, which placed limitations on my ability to be physically active.

I had been following a starch-based vegan diet. I had lost some weight, but I always felt hungry. I constantly thought about the next meal and had to carefully count calories in order to avoid overeating. My skin looked pale and was extremely dry. I then discovered and began following Dr. Fuhrman's nutritarian program. I am now vibrant, colorful, and alive—functioning every day at my very best and enjoying life to the fullest! I enjoy the food that I eat now, and I love the fact that I can eat this way, feel great, and stay at an ideal weight. I now enjoy an active life and have the energy to do so much more than I ever did before.

I love knowing that I'm in control of my health destiny, and that I'm not doomed to suffer and die from chronic diseases that plague many Americans. It doesn't matter how many times you've tried and failed in the past—anyone can do this.

High saturated fat and the heme iron contents of red meat have also been demonstrated to increase the risk of cardiovascular disease. Saturated fats are known to elevate total cholesterol and LDL levels, and excess iron is associated with oxidative stress, which promotes atherosclerosis.[30] Interestingly, one of the mechanisms by which the combination of saturated fat and red meat increases disease risk is that saturated fat intake facilitates the absorption of the heme iron. Heme iron and saturated fat can work synergistically to oxidize cholesterol, increasing the small oxidized LDL particles that are the most dangerous. Your body can turn down the absorption of non-heme iron (from plant foods) if it's not currently in need of iron, but it absorbs the heme iron found in animal foods whether it needs iron or not. Iron is an essential mineral that transports oxygen in the blood and has many other crucial functions, but an excess of iron leads to free radical damage, which increases your susceptibility to chronic diseases, especially those with an oxidative stress component such as heart disease and stroke.[31] A recent meta-analysis further confirmed the link between red and processed meat and the substantial increased risk of ischemic stroke.[32] Heme iron can also promote the peroxidation of dietary fat, even salad oils, so a diet rich in red meat along with vegetable oil and salad oil can increase free radical damage from the oil.

Several studies have found that a higher intake of meat and heme iron is also linked to high blood pressure, while intake of high non-heme iron (from plant foods) is associated with low blood pressure.[33]

Wait, there is more fascinating new research that has revealed another mechanism by which red and white meat increases cardiovascular risk—by modulating the species of bacteria that populate our digestive tract. What we eat determines which species of bacteria thrive in our guts. Healthful, fiber-rich plant foods provide an energy source ("prebiotics") for beneficial bacteria to grow.[34] For example, carnitine, an amino acid abundant in animal products, is barely present in plant foods, if at all. The human body can produce adequate amounts of carnitine from other amino acids such as lysine and methionine. (Cells require carnitine to transport fatty acid.) The mechanism was first discovered in mice, when scientists found that carnitine in the diet was metabolized by intestinal bacteria, producing trimethylamine-N-oxide (TMAO). This is a substance previously shown to contribute to atherosclerotic plaque development by slowing the removal of cholesterol from the arterial wall. Then when analyzing the blood levels of carnitine and TMAO in human subjects, these same scientists found that high levels of these two substances combined to increase the likelihood of cardiovascular disease or cardiovascular events such as heart attack and stroke. When they gave humans carnitine supplements, those who were omnivores produced far more TMAO than vegans and vegetarians. In addition, the species of gut bacteria in omnivores differed from the species found in vegetarians and vegans. These results suggest that regularly eating meat promotes the growth of gut bacteria that can metabolize carnitine into a heart disease–promoting substance.[35]

Such results suggest that those of us who regularly consume a healthful diet of mostly whole plant foods have a healthier microbial profile and are therefore less susceptible to the problems associated with carnitine. An overwhelming amount of evidence now links meat to cancer and premature death, leaving no doubt that even pasture-raised meat and meat products should generally be avoided or minimized in the diet.[36] If you still want to eat meat, you should eat it as if it were a condiment; that is, only eat it a few times a week and in small amounts. Remember to choose the most natural and cleanest sources of meat possible: grass-fed meats, wild fish, and naturally raised, hormone-free poultry. And avoid dangerous processed meats, barbecued meats, lunch meats, bacon, hot dogs, and any pickled, darkened, or blackened animal products.

Eat Safely, Wisely, and Well

Sure, we need enough protein for muscle growth and maintenance and protection against age-related skeletal decline, but this need is best met by including protein-rich plant proteins into your diet, most notably greens, beans, and seeds. Green vegetables, beans and other legumes, and seeds are rich in plant protein and have cancer-preventive, not cancer-promoting, properties. For optimal cancer protection, you should get the vast majority of your calories from vegetables, beans, fruits, whole grains, nuts, and seeds (see Table 1 on page 50).

All animal products, including meat, fish, and dairy, are low or completely lacking in the nutrients that protect us against cancer and heart attacks: fiber, antioxidants, and hundreds of phytochemicals. So many people have been indoctrinated to think that animal protein is needed or superior to plant protein, when the opposite is true.

In the past, I have recommended eggs as the cleanest source of animal protein. But recent studies have forced me to reconsider eggs as a recommended animal product option for overweight individuals. These studies have established that a high consumption of eggs can lead to diabetes, heart disease, and prostate cancer. Eggs are high in cholesterol, and high cholesterol impairs your body's glucose tolerance and pancreatic function, which can lead to diabetes, and for people who already have diabetes, to premature death. The Physicians' Health Study, for example, reported a 23 percent increased death rate from those eating more than one egg a day.[37] These negative effects were substantially higher in diabetics. The Health Professionals Follow-up Study found that people who ate more than one egg per week substantially increased their risk of developing diabetes. People who ate more than seven eggs a week increased this risk by 58 percent.[38] If an individual already had diabetes, death rates doubled if that person consumed more than seven eggs a week. Similarly, a Greek study of diabetics reported a fivefold increase in cardiovascular death for people who ate at least one egg per day.[39]

Eggs are also particularly rich in choline, which, like cholesterol, is highly concentrated in prostate cancer cells.[40] A 2011 study that followed 27,607 men from 1994 to 2008 found that the ones who consumed two and a half or more eggs per week had an 81 percent increased risk of prostate cancer compared with men who consumed less than half an egg per week.[41] The Health Professionals Follow-up Study, which looked at the egg consumption of 47,896 men, corroborated this. Men in the highest quintile of choline intake had a 70 percent increased risk of prostate cancer.[42]

Other studies have found choline to be involved in cancer growth and progression.[43] For example, increased choline intake was associated with a higher risk of colorectal adenomas in the highly respected Nurses' Health Study.[44] A 2012 study measured the correlation between egg yolk consumption and carotid artery plaque in more than twelve hundred individuals. The plaque inside blood vessels increased proportionately to the number of egg yolks consumed. For those with the highest egg consumption, the results were almost as bad as they would have been if the study subjects had been smokers.[45] Individuals who ate the most eggs yolks, averaging about four per week, exhibited two-thirds the plaque formation in their carotid arteries as a person who smoked a pack a day for forty years! Study after study continues to show that egg yolks aren't as harmless as advertised, or as generally believed. They are especially risky for overweight people with prediabetes or diabetes.

I want you to stop worrying about consuming enough protein. Almost all Americans get enough daily protein. In fact, the average American consumes more than 100 grams of protein each day, about 50 percent more than the recommended daily amount. You don't need to rely on animal products for protein. Almost any assortment of vegetables, beans, whole grains, seeds, and nuts will supply about 40 grams of protein per 1,000 calories. This means that a typical 2,000-calorie diet provides us about 80 grams of protein—much more than what we need.

I hope you realize now that our common concern ingrained in us in our childhood about getting sufficient protein was an error. The main concern should be about not getting too much. When we meet our needs for calories with natural plant foods, we automatically get sufficient protein—without even trying.

The only way even a vegan diet could be deficient in protein is if the diet were composed of almost all fruit, refined grains, and junk food. Vegetables, whole grains, beans, nuts, and seeds all have adequate amounts of protein. It's exceedingly rare that an individual has unique needs that necessitate his or her eating animal products to get more protein, and when that does occur, a very small amount of animal product suffices. Generally, other high-protein plant foods can be substituted, even for individuals who require more protein.

Beans, hemp seeds, Mediterranean pine nuts, sunflower seeds, and soybeans (including tempeh, tofu, and bean pasta) can be used to enhance the protein content of a diet for athletes and people with higher protein needs without going crazy with animal products. Even professional athletes can get sufficient protein when eating a properly designed vegan diet, once they know how to utilize those high-protein plant foods.

The only nutrients lacking in a vegan diet are vitamin B_{12} and the long-chain omega-3 fatty acids EPA and DHA. One should also consider supplementation with iodine and vitamin D, depending on one's exposure to sunshine and consumption of seaweed for iodine. The amount of zinc might be somewhat suboptimal with a vegan diet because of zinc binding by phytates in plants, but otherwise, animal products don't provide anything that you can't get in a safer package— from consuming plant foods. So eat less animal products—consider hardly eating them at all—for the best health and then supplement wisely and conservatively to make up for any insufficiencies.

Beware of Salmon

Most fish today is raised in fish farms, and they could be the most polluted foods we eat. Consider salmon, once thought to be a healthy food choice because of its omega-3 fatty acid content. But the vast majority of salmon sold in grocery stores and restaurants today is commercial farmed-raised salmon, which has been found to contain levels of toxins roughly ten times worse than the levels found in most commercial beef.[46] According to the U.S. Environmental Protection Agency's guidelines for exposure to the toxic chemical compound dioxin, even one meal of salmon a month can pose unacceptable cancer risks. Researchers analyzed seven hundred farmed and wild salmon samples from eight major regions around the world sold in North America and Europe and found dangerous levels of PCBs, dioxins, and the insecticides dieldrin and toxaphene in the farmed salmon.

The difference between the concentrations of contaminants found in farmed and wild salmon is most likely a result of the fishes' diets. Wild salmon eat a large variety of aquatic organisms such as krill, zooplankton, and small fish; but farmed salmon primarily consume a formulated high-fat feed of other fish ground into fishmeal mixed with fish oil. This encourages rapid growth. As far back as 2003, the National Academy of Sciences noted problems with this fishmeal diet and called for the reduction of dioxin exposure in farmed fish.

Researchers have also documented high levels of marine pollution coming from salmon farms due to the release of large quantities of waste, antibiotics, and other chemicals generated during salmon farming. Everyone assumes that eating salmon is healthy, and that's why it has become so popular. But the reality is that farm-raised salmon is one of the most cancer-promoting foods we can eat. If you eat even a little fish, you should choose wild-caught fish from cleaner parts of the ocean or from safe fish farms known to have high-quality standards in the industry.

A Nutritarian Lifestyle Followed for Life

With the right food as the catalyst, your body will heal itself. Health, longevity, and weight loss are all products of healthy foods such as greens and other colorful vegetables, fruits, beans, nuts, and seeds. Vegetables and other nutrient-rich produce will fill you up, crowd out unhealthy food choices, encourage good bowel function, flood the body with needed antioxidants and immune-supporting phytochemicals, fuel the growth of beneficial flora in your stomach and bowels, and create a favorable hormonal balance that reduces fat storage and prevents cancer.

In fact, I encourage you to eat a larger volume of high-nutrient plants, including big salads and lots of tomato, onion, raw and cooked greens, and cooked mushrooms. Eat large portions of healthy food, prepared deliciously, which effectively blunts your appetite for more concentrated calories and unhealthful food choices. Not only will you look and feel great, but you can prevent heart disease, cancer, and other deadly maladies. The focus is on eating more of the right foods—foods that can save your life.

Over the past twenty years, I have counseled thousands of people in my medical practice, over the Internet, and at speaking events and weeklong "Getaways" or "Immersions." Most of these folks come to me unhappy, sick, and overweight, having tried every dietary craze without success. Most have said to me, "I just can't lose weight no matter what I do." My nutritarian approach to eating has helped so many of these people lose their excess weight and keep it off permanently. They were able to live up to their full health potential, all while learning to prefer this way of eating over their old diets. Thousands of individuals are now living examples of the success of this approach; they would never even consider eating any other way—ever. They finally have reached the End of Dieting.

CHAPTER SIX

The Plan

The goal is to structure a balanced life for yourself that combines work, eating, shopping, food preparation, gardening, family time, exercise, social pleasures, and entertainment—a life that is enjoyable, varied, keeps you feeling well and emotionally satisfied but also protects you, your family, and our world. This is all about how to live for life—a good life! It just takes a little more effort for some to get there, but it is worth the trip.

Rather than focusing on all the foods you *can't* eat, enjoy all the foods that you *can* eat in unlimited quantities. Be determined to get though the threshold of unhealthy food cravings. Once the cravings for unhealthy foods decrease and your taste buds change, the natural desire for nutrient-rich foods will take precedence. You'll no longer feel deprived, and eating will become more enjoyable and pleasurable than ever before.

Don't let one little slipup derail you on your quest for good health. Get right back on the program with the next meal (not the next day).

Six Basic Guidelines for the Nutritarian Diet Style

Everybody can do this, and here's the plan. But remember: These are just general guidelines; you don't have to follow them precisely. For example, you can go above or below the general serving recommendations depending on your height and degree of physical activity or exercise. A world-class athlete may need triple the calories of a sedentary office worker.

To call yourself a nutritarian, follow these six basic guidelines:

1. Eat a large salad every day as your main dish.
This salad should include lettuce, tomatoes, shredded onion, and at least one shredded raw cruciferous vegetable, such as chopped kale, red cabbage, nappa cabbage, arugula, watercress, or baby bok choy.

Use a variety of greens, including romaine, mixed greens, mesclun mix, arugula, baby spinach, Boston lettuce, and watercress. For added veggies, choose from red and green bell peppers, cucumbers, carrots, bean sprouts, shredded red or green cabbage, chopped white and red onions, lightly sautéed mushrooms, lightly steamed and sliced zucchini, raw and lightly steamed beets and carrots, snow peas, broccoli, cauliflower, and radishes. I often add some frozen peas and beans to my salads too.

Add a healthy dressing (one that is nut and seed based), such as my tomato sauce–based Russian Fig Dressing on page 221, which blends almonds and sunflower seeds with a dark vinegar and a fig or a few currants or raisins.

I usually make a huge salad, share it with family members, and have enough left over for later in the day or the next day.

> Remember, for superior health, the green salad
> is the main dish, not the side dish.

2. Eat at least a half cup, but preferably closer to 1 cup, of beans a day.

This means eating a bean burger, a bean loaf, or a veggie-bean soup or putting beans on your salad or in a stew or chili in the evening. In our household, we almost always make a giant pot of veggie bean soup once a week. After eating the soup that day, I portion it into eight containers and refrigerate or freeze it so I can take it to work with me or use it when I need it. Quick tip: Use some of the soup you made as a unique salad dressing base by adding some flavored vinegar and nuts. Blend in a high-powered blender until smooth.

3. Eat one large (double-size) serving of lightly steamed green vegetables a day.

This means a bowl of asparagus, chopped kale with a delicious mushroom/onion sauce, green beans, steamed zucchini, bok choy, artichokes, cabbage, or collard greens. Don't overcook greens; thirteen minutes of steaming is plenty. The longer you cook them, the more micronutrients you burn off, which wastes the effects of phytochemicals. Green vegetables need to be fully chewed (to the consistency of nearly liquid in your mouth) for you to fully benefit from their anti-cancer phytonutrients.

4. Eat at least 1 ounce of nuts and seeds per day if you're female and at least 1.5 ounces of nuts and seeds per day if you're male.

Remember, don't use nuts and seeds as snacks. They are the healthiest way to take in fat with meals and demonstrate a powerful effect on extending the human lifespan. The fat from nuts and seeds, when eaten with vegetables, increases the phytochemical absorption from those veggies. That's why I typically recommend that nuts and seeds be part of your salad dressing, too. Also, at least half of this intake should be from walnuts, hemp seeds, chia seeds, flaxseeds, and sesame seeds because they have unique protective properties, such as lignans and omega-3 fatty acids.

Eating 3 to 4 ounces of nuts and seeds a day isn't too much if you're active and slim. There's no problem with eating even more than 4 ounces of nuts and seeds per day if you're an avid exerciser or athlete who needs the calories. I have worked with professional football players and Olympic skiers who follow this diet style; obviously, they need lots more seeds and nuts, and other food too.

Eat nuts and seeds raw, or just lightly toasted, because the roasting process alters their beneficial fats. Commercially packaged nuts and seeds are also frequently cooked in oil and are heavily salted. If you want to add some flavor, lightly toast seeds and nuts in a toaster oven on one low toasting cycle. This doesn't deplete their beneficial properties. Don't toast to the point of dark browning, however, as this can cause carcinogenic compounds called acrylamides to be formed. You can also bake them in a 250°F oven for about fifteen minutes, or until very lightly browned.

5. Eat mushrooms and onions every day.

Both mushrooms and onions have powerful anticancer benefits. Mushrooms are better eaten cooked because some mushrooms contain a mild carcinogen called agaritine. It is gassed off during cooking. Only the *Agaricus* genus of mushrooms—which includes the common white, brown, button, cremini, and portobello mushrooms—contains agaritine. Shiitake, chanterelle, enoki, morel, oyster, and straw mushrooms belong to different genera that don't contain agaritine. But they should also be cooked to reduce the risk of any potential contamination with microbes. It's still not entirely clear whether agaritine is a health risk, but play it safe and cook most of your mushrooms with your other vegetables, or water-sauté them in a wok or other pan. Keep a container of cooked mushrooms in your fridge to add to salads and vegetable dishes regularly.

6. Eat three fresh fruits a day.

Fresh fruits aren't just nutritious and delicious, they also protect against disease. The phytochemicals in fruits have anticancer effects, and berries have even been shown to protect the brain from dementia in later life. Try to eat one serving of berries or pomegranate a day as part of your total fruit intake. When eaten with a meal, vegetables dilute and slow your body's absorption of glucose and fructose, so it's best to eat fruit as part of your vegetable-based meal, either mixed in with your salad or as a dessert. If you're physically active, you can certainly eat more than three fruits a day, but it's still best to avoid fruit juice and too much dried fruit, such as dates, raisins, figs, and prunes, because they are calorically dense and could elevate your blood sugar if you eat them in large amounts. When making a recipe or dessert that contains dried fruit for flavor and sweetness, limit the amount to 2 tablespoons per serving. That means one Medjool date or two Deglet Noor dates per dessert serving; otherwise, you could be consuming too much simple sugar.

That's it. Six simple guidelines to follow. That's not so difficult to do, is it? Can you imagine what would happen if everyone in the United States followed these guidelines?

- We would stop the healthcare crisis in its tracks and save billions of dollars on medical expenses.

- We would save millions of lives from premature death.

- We would reduce rates of heart disease, stroke, dementia, and cancer by more than 80 percent.

- We would have less crime, and a more successful, intelligent, and productive workforce.

- We would have many fewer people in nursing homes, fewer stroke victims, and fewer elderly people suffering from dementia and unable to enjoy life.

NUTRITARIAN DAILY CHECKLIST

(Make copies of this chart and check off each point each day.)

☐ Eat a large salad as the main dish for at least one meal.

☐ Eat at least a half cup, but preferably closer to 1 cup, of beans.

☐ Eat one large (double-size) serving of steamed green vegetables.

☐ Eat at least 1 ounce of nuts and seeds if you're female and at least 1.5 ounces of nuts and seeds if you're male. Half of them should be walnuts, hemp seeds, chia seeds, flaxseeds, or sesame seeds.

☐ Eat some cooked mushrooms and raw and cooked onions.

☐ Eat at least three fresh fruits.

The Simple End of Dieting Plan

Many people have contacted me about wanting a simple plan without fancy recipes. They don't have the time to spend all day in the kitchen. They live in a fast-food world, holding down two jobs or being busy with their families—or both. "I can't spend half my week in the kitchen," they tell me, "chopping vegetables and putting together complicated recipes."

Even if this is you, you can still do this. Remember: No obstacles, no excuses. Find a way; there's always a solution to protect your life. There are many ways to make this work. For instance, you could shop and cook one evening a week and one weekend morning and then prepare all your food for the week.

You can get started by following this simple version of my nutrient-dense eating style that doesn't entail much in the way of cooking and preparation. You don't have to prepare extensive and detailed recipes. Indeed, the purpose of this book is to help you end all obstacles and even the smallest source of contention, turning every person who touches its pages into a nutritarian. Use this sample core menu to devise your own meals, or follow the sample menu plans toward the end of this chapter.

Simple Core Menu

Breakfast

Intact grain, such as steel-cut oats, or old-fashioned oats with
some ground flaxseeds, hemp seeds, or chia seeds added.

Or a slice of 100 percent whole grain bread with nut butter (and
banana).

A serving of fresh or frozen fruit.

Consider making some quick homemade Hemp Almond Milk, which
takes just two minutes with a high-powered blender. See page 208.

Lunch

Huge salad with a nut/seed-based dressing (see pages 217–223 for
lots of options, or Table 17 for commercial dressings).

Bowl of vegetable bean soup (see pages 234–240 for recipes or
Tables 15–16 for prepared soups).

One fresh fruit.

Dinner

Salad or raw veggies with a bean-, nut-, or vegetable-based dip.

Simple cooked vegetable-based entrée.

Include in your entrée green vegetables as well as some nutrient-
dense nongreen vegetables such as tomatoes, eggplant, onions, mushrooms, cauliflower, or peppers. Great choices are steamed or water-
sautéed green vegetables served on top of whole grain black or wild
rice, bean pasta or squash, mushroom-bean burgers, tofu/tempeh chili,
or water-sautéed kale with mushrooms, onions, and beans.

Frozen fruit dessert.

ARE YOUR GRAINS INTACT?

What are intact grains? They are grains that are still in their original form—that is, the outer bran layer, the middle layer (or endosperm), and the inner germ layer of the grain remain intact. Intact grains have a better nutritional profile and a lower glycemic index than grains that have been refined. Intact grains include wild and black rice, steel-cut oats, bulgur wheat, wheat berries, and hulled barley (also known as barley groats, scotch barley, or pot barley).

To make my favorite nutritarian breakfast, combine an intact grain, such as steel-cut oats, with nondairy milk (such as soy or almond milk) and soak overnight. In the morning, mix in fruit (fresh or frozen) and ground flaxseed or chia seeds.

Meat Lovers Rejoice

I can make this same Simple Core Menu favorable for all the dyed-in-the-wool meat eaters who don't want to give up the taste of meat. You can get almost the same lifespan and health benefits as a vegan nutritarian by using a small amount of animal product to flavor your veggie burger, chili, or soup. By mixing just a small amount (about 1 ounce per serving) of meat into my mushroom-bean burgers (see Meat-Lover's Beef, Bean, and Mushroom Burgers, page 267), for example, you have healthful, flavorful burgers that taste better than the typical all-beef patty, with only one-fifth the amount of meat—barely 1 ounce of animal products—for the entire day. This is almost an insignificant amount. You can call it the Soup, Salad, and Burger diet!

Otherwise, limit animal products served in a larger portion (3–5 ounces) to just once a week. This keeps the total number of ounces of animal products per week to less than 10 ounces. Then the six other days when you eat only 1–2 ounces won't be enough to significantly increase IGF-1 levels over baseline for most people.

Still, if you're using animal products in your diet, it might be wise to have your doctor check your IGF-1 level to make sure it's less than

150 nanograms per milliliter. If it isn't, you should strongly consider reducing, or eliminating, the animal products in your diet, and, of course, be careful with your intake of sweets.

Here are my suggestions if you still want to include the flavor of animal products in your diet:

1. Eat a maximum of 1.5 ounces of meat a day if you're female and only 2.5 ounces if you're male as a flavoring agent in a recipe or dish.

2. Eat only 2.5 ounces if you're female and 3.5 ounces if you're male once a day, but then make the next day completely vegan so your weekly intake remains less than 10 ounces (females) or 16 ounces (males).

3. If you have a bigger serving, such as 5–7 ounces, then have that amount only once weekly or less.

As a general rule, try to keep your calories from animal products below 5 percent of your total daily caloric intake. Since a reasonable number of daily calories is 1,600 for women and 2,400 for men, 5 percent of calories a day equals about 80 calories for women and 120 for men. Or about 560 calories a week for women and about 840 calories a week for men. This would limit your exposure to IGF-1 and keep your caloric intake of animal products in line with that of the people from the longest-lived societies around the world.

I should be clear. I am not recommending that most people consume animal products. Available evidence demonstrates that a vegan diet with the right supplements is, for most people, still the most likely path to maximizing lifespan. Of course, we're not all robots. Some people thrive better with a small amount of animal products. For those of you who don't want to go completely vegan nutritarian, this option is a healthy way to continue to enjoy the flavor of animal products without raising IGF-1 to levels that promote cancer.

Keep It Simple

It's simple to eat this way without hours and hours of food preparation. For instance, make a healthy salad dressing every Wednesday and Saturday and eat that dressing for three days. (See pages 217 to 223 for easy-to-make basic dressings.) Alternatively, if you're on the go, you can buy one of my healthy salad dressings to make your life easier. Table 17, on pages 198–199, lists my Dr. Fuhrman dressings as well as other brands that may be viable options for you. You can even mix a less healthy dressing in with one of mine or with a little tomato paste or tomato sauce to make something work for you.

Once or twice a week, make a giant pot of vegetable bean soup and use that soup for several days to limit cooking chores. Alternatively, purchase one of my healthy soups to make your life easier; see Tables 15 and 16 for easy soup options. I have worked hard with my executive team in New Jersey to produce a line of super-healthful soups and salad dressings that make the no-time-to-cook obstacles no longer an issue. For busy people this can be predominantly a soup and salad diet style, so if you have the salad dressing and the soup readily available, it becomes simple to fit healthy food preparation and eating into your busy lifestyle.

Chapter 7 includes a variety of my favorite recipes. Many are quick and simple to prepare. As the nutritarian eating style becomes a way of life for you, sample these recipes, find your favorites, and include them regularly in your daily menus.

I Hate to Cook

You hate to cook? Not a problem. With just a few cartons of soup, a few salad dressings, some fresh and frozen fruits and vegetables, and some nuts and seeds and maybe some oats, you can organize your weekly menus without fuss.

Think about the food you need to eat in one day. Three or four fresh or frozen fruits. One carton or one can of soup, or the equivalent amount of homemade soup. A quarter cup of salad dressing on your huge lunch salad. And about 2 cups of steamed or frozen green vegetables for dinner. Open a bag and defrost some frozen peas, snow pea pods, Brussels sprouts, frozen artichokes, or broccoli and then pour some dressing or make one of my easy dips. It doesn't need to be complicated.

It's Too Expensive

People sometimes say that they can't afford to eat this way—that fresh fruits and vegetables are too expensive. But this doesn't have to be true. Following a nutritarian diet style doesn't have to cost any more than a diet based on meat and highly processed foods. Take a look at the cost of a typical daily standard American diet meal compared with a nutritarian one.

Standard American Diet: Menu Cost, $16.07

Breakfast
Bagel with cream cheese
Orange juice
Coffee

Lunch
Fast-food cheeseburgers (two of them), French fries, and a soda

Snack
Two chocolate chip cookies with milk

Dinner

Mixed greens salad with tomato and purchased ranch dressing

Frozen lasagna

Vanilla ice cream

Iced tea

NUTRITION FACTS FOR THIS MENU: CALORIES 2,692; PROTEIN 78g; CARBOHY-DRATES 344g; TOTAL FAT 115g; SATURATED FAT 46g; SODIUM 3,686mg; FIBER 21g; BETA-CAROTENE 826mcg; VITAMIN C 207mg; CALCIUM 1,362mg; IRON 17mg; FO-LATE 591mcg; MAGNESIUM 261mg; ZINC 11.6mg; SELENIUM 93mcg

PROTEIN 11.4 percent; CARBOHYDRATE 50.5 percent; TOTAL FAT 38.1 percent

Nutritarian Diet:
Menu Cost, $14.50

Breakfast

Oatmeal with blueberries and chia seeds

Hemp Almond Milk (1 cup)

Lunch

Salad of mixed greens with tomato, bell pepper, red onion, and
   sunflower seeds and purchased low-sodium, no-oil dressing

Homemade vegetable bean soup

Apple

Dinner

Raw veggies—such as carrots, bell pepper, radishes, fennel, snow
   peas, cherry tomatoes, and cucumber—dipped in purchased
   dressing

Mushroom-bean burgers on whole grain pita bread with lettuce,
   tomato, and red onion

Fruit sorbet

NUTRITION FACTS FOR THIS MENU: CALORIES 1,897; PROTEIN 65g; CARBOHY-DRATES 275g; TOTAL FAT 75g; SATURATED FAT 8g; SODIUM 487mg; FIBER 57g; BETA-

CAROTENE 28,965mcg; VITAMIN C 333mg; CALCIUM 865mg; IRON 22.1mg; FOLATE 973mcg; MAGNESIUM 864mg; ZINC 15.2mg; SELENIUM 85mcg

PROTEIN 12.8 percent; CARBOHYDRATE 54.1 percent; TOTAL FAT 33.0 percent

A nutritarian diet style can save your life and save you money. You are what you eat, so you might as well spend your money on quality food. Think about this. We spend ten times as much on medical care today than we did seventy years ago but only about one-quarter as much on food as a percentage of our take-home pay. We lowered the quality of our diets, so now we have to pay so much more for medical care, and we are so sickly that it is harder to afford to buy fresh food anymore.

Twelve Helpful Tips

1. The secret weight-loss food is eggplant.

Eggplants have only 20 calories per cup. Do you have 20 pounds to lose? One hundred? Then try eating more food for once, rather than less. More eggplant, more cauliflower, more green vegetables with mushrooms and onions, more salad, more roasted peppers, and more stewed tomatoes and garlic.

Yesterday, I baked a fresh eggplant in the oven with the skin on at 360°F for forty minutes. I didn't do anything except put the eggplant in the oven and turn the oven on. Then I heated a frying pan and added a couple of cups of finely chopped onion, tossing and mixing them with a wooden spoon until they glistened and had a slight tan. I took out the cooked eggplant, sliced it in half, turned it skin-side up (meaty center down), and, using a dish towel, squeezed the skin off, leaving the soft cooked center on the plate. I mixed in the onions, added a tablespoon of Ceylon cinnamon, and it was done. (Sometimes I add some currants and chopped raw onion.)

Not only did I have a great dish, but I had leftovers for the next day—and it was delicious cold. After eating my big salad and the eggplant, and a box of raspberries for dessert, I was too full to eat another bite. The next morning, I was starving because my dinner, which had made me feel so full, was so low in calories that I was hungry again as soon as I woke up. Get it? Getting hungry can be fun. Foods taste better, and since you can eat whenever you want—and as much as you want—you are never dieting. You'll gravitate to and then stay at your ideal weight forever.

2. Eat more of the foods that promote weight loss.

These foods are unlimited, and you can eat as much of them as you want. The more you eat, the better—within reason; you should never eat until you feel uncomfortable. You actually should never even recognize that you have a stomach. Stop eating when you feel satisfied; stop eating if you start to feel full. Never overeat; never eat until you're "stuffed." It's still possible, though, to eat as much food as is reasonable. Here's a list of the foods that are most favorable to weight loss. Eat lots of them if you have a significant amount of weight to lose.

> *All raw vegetables*—Not only are vegetables naturally low in calories, but when you eat them raw, more of the calories stay bound to the fiber and pass through your body without absorption. Even raw carrots are a weight-loss-friendly food.

> *All green vegetables*—If they are the color green, go for it. Green vegetables are not just low in caloric density, they are super high in micronutrient density too.

> *Nonstarchy, nongreen cooked vegetables*—Include tomatoes, onions, mushrooms, cauliflower, eggplant, and red peppers in your diet.

3. Use a low-calorie salsa or hummus as a dressing or dip.

You might find that a dressing or dip makes it easier to enjoy lots of the raw vegetables that are so healthful and such an important part of the natural human diet. Tomatoes, carrot sticks, fennel bulbs, snow pea pods, raw peas, raw string beans, raw broccoli, raw cauliflower, even strips of kohlrabi, cabbage, and radish taste great raw with a nice dip.

Hummus is a great dip and easy to make. All you have to do is blend some cooked, boxed, or canned chickpeas with unhulled sesame seeds, scallions, and roasted garlic. Check out the Roasted Eggplant Hummus on page 224.

A technique I frequently use when cooking is to roast an entire bulb of garlic and squeeze out the roasted "paste" that is formed. I then mix that in a recipe along with one clove of crushed raw garlic. When you don't use salt or oil for flavoring, roasted garlic, stewed or water-sautéed onion, lemon, and gourmet flavored vinegars add lots of flavor.

A salsa is easy to make too. Just chop some plum tomatoes with scallions, add a touch of chopped chili pepper if desired, add a tablespoon of almond butter and some soft red beans from a box, mix it all together, add some dried currants, and you have a great dip that will last for days. Check out some of my favorite salsa recipes on pages 225 and 226.

4. Have a steamed green vegetable every night for dinner.

Steaming a veggie is quick and easy. You only need a steamer pot with a lid or a steamer basket to place in a pot with a lid. Alternatively, you can improvise a steamer by placing in the bottom of a pot a few stalks of celery or the outer leaves of a head of lettuce or cabbage that you were going to discard. Add a small amount of water, cover, and cook for the appropriate length of time.

Don't steam vegetables until they're very soft. At that point, the water has turned green and you've washed away half of the water-soluble nutrients. The trick is to stop steaming when the vegetables have just started to become tender and still retain some firmness. Table 13 shows the steaming times I find work best. Boil water in a pot with a tight lid first, then add the vegetables, cover, and start your timer. These times assume the artichokes have been cut in half and prepped and the cabbage and broccoli stems have been sliced. Ready, set, go!

TABLE 13. VEGETABLE STEAMING TIMES

VEGETABLE	TIME
Artichokes	18 minutes
Asparagus	13 minutes
Bok choy	10 minutes
Broccoli	13 minutes
Brussels sprouts	13 minutes
Cabbage	13 minutes
Kale, collards, Swiss chard	10 minutes
Snow peas	10 minutes
String beans	13 minutes
Zucchini	13 minutes

Anatomy of an Artichoke

Thorn—sharp barbs at the tip of each leaf

Outer leaves—tough and fibrous; small pith where leaf attaches is the only edible part

Inner leaves—more tender than outer leaves; edible in young artichoke hearts or quarters

Heart—the meaty, succulent center

Choke—fine, fuzzy, hair-like filaments

Stem—stringy outer layer, meaty center

Artichoke Cross Section

Tips for Preparing Artichokes

To cook an artichoke, slice 1 inch off the tip. Cut off about ½ inch or less of the very bottom piece of the stem to expose the fresh green bottom, keeping the remaining stem attached. Then, using a large, sharp knife, slice the artichoke in half lengthwise. Once sliced in half, you can see the fuzzy inedible choke part. Use a small, pointed knife to cut a deep half-moon-shaped incision where the heart meets the choke. Scoop out and discard the fibrous and hairy choke from the center of each half. Place the artichoke in a steamer basket over several inches of water. Bring the water to a boil, cover, and steam for eighteen minutes. Set the artichoke aside until it's cool enough to handle.

To eat, peel off the outer leaves one at a time. Tightly grip the outer end of the leaf, place the opposite end in your mouth, and pull through your teeth to remove the soft, pulpy, delicious portion of the leaf. You can also scrape off the edible portion with a butter knife. Then you can eat it plain or prepare a healthful dip or dressing to use as a dip. Continue until all the leaves are removed. Cut the remaining heart into pieces and enjoy!

Tip for Preparing Broccoli

Cut off the stems from the florets and cut them in quarters, lengthwise, first in half and then in half again. Steam the cut stems and florets for about thirteen minutes. Or, if you like the stems more tender, put them in the pot to steam for two minutes and then add the florets for thirteen minutes more.

---

5. Make bean dinner loaves and fruity desserts.

Make a bean dinner loaf by mixing mashed cooked or canned white beans, onions, and mushrooms; add ground marjoram, nutritional yeast, and agar, and then bake. Serve it hot or cold. Check out the Vegetable Chickpea Loaf recipe on page 256.

Agar, a vegetarian gelatin made from seaweed, is the secret to this loaf. It's sold in health food stores in both flake and powder forms and can be used as a thickening agent in a variety of recipes.

To make a gelatin fruit dessert, combine 1 tablespoon of agar powder and 1 cup of water. Bring the water to a boil, remove from the heat, and stir to dissolve the agar completely. Mix in the desired ingredients, such as fresh fruit and a small amount of dried fruit chopped and soaked in almond or hemp milk. Add both the dried fruit and the thickened soaking milk. Mix well and then cool until it firms up. For another simple yet elegant dessert, try the Strawberry Panna Cotta on page 282.

6. Enhance flavors.

Your taste buds may be used to a lot of salt, so at first, this new eating routine may seem a little bland. This will change after a few weeks, however, and then you'll experience and enjoy the real taste of food. Your taste muscle will continue to improve for months, as your health improves and you remain off salt and sweeteners. In the meantime, there are many ways to healthfully flavor your meals.

Roast garlic. Roasted garlic is milder, richer, and sweeter than raw garlic. You can use it in salad dressings, dips, soups, and vegetable dishes. Roast unpeeled garlic in a 350°F oven for twenty-five minutes or until soft. When cool, remove the skins and add the paste to whatever you like. I recommend having a small glass jar of roasted garlic in the fridge at all times to mash into various dishes and dressings.

Use tomato paste. Tomato paste consists of tomatoes that have been cooked for several hours and reduced to a thick, red concentrate before being strained. You can use it to flavor, thicken, and color soups, stews, and other vegetable dishes. Be careful when choosing tomato products. Many metal cans are lined with a BPA-containing resin. Since tomatoes are acidic, a significant amount of BPA (bisphenol-A) could leach into the food. BPA is a chemical linked to a number of negative health effects. Look for tomato paste and other tomato products packaged in materials that do not contain BPA, such as glass or cartons. Some manufacturers are utilizing or may utilize another BPA-free epoxy to line their cans, which certainly is an improvement, but I still prefer to purchase tomato products in glass or cartons so there is no concern about the acidity of the tomatoes reacting with the lining.

Use dried (not sun-dried) tomatoes. Dried or dehydrated tomatoes add flavor and nutritional value to many recipes. You can add them directly to soups and stew, or soak them in water to cover for thirty to sixty minutes and then add them to salads. Include the soaking water in your recipes, as it contains some of the nutrients from the tomatoes. Salt and sulfites are added to most sun-dried tomatoes to preserve them during the extended drying process. Sulfites are a preservative and enhance color, but some people are sensitive to them and respond with adverse reactions. Look for unsulfured and unsalted dried tomatoes that have been hot air dried, not sun dried. The faster drying time allows them to be processed without preservatives.

Soak dried fruits and currants. Small amounts of dried fruit, such as raisins, currants, prunes, apricots, or figs, add sweetness to salads and vegetable dishes. Soak dried fruit in enough hot water to cover until soft (about thirty minutes), or soak in water or soy or hemp milk overnight. Soaking softens the fruit and improves the texture and flavor. If possible, incorporate the soaking liquid into your recipe to obtain nutrients and flavor that may have leached into the water.

Roast peppers. Roasting peppers imparts a subtle smokiness to the peppers while bringing out their sweet flavor. Roasted peppers are great in Mexican-inspired dishes, such as vegetable fajitas, roasted red pepper dip, and chili. They're great in salads, too. Roast peppers by placing them on a rimmed baking pan in a 375°F oven for fifty to sixty minutes, turning every twenty minutes, until the peppers are evenly browned and soft. Let them cool, and then peel them and remove the seeds.

Toast nuts and seeds. Nuts and seeds are delicious raw, but lightly toasting them brings out their flavor and makes them crunchy. Toasted almonds, sesame seeds, and pine nuts add flavor to salads and can be sprinkled on soups or hot vegetable dishes. To toast nuts or seeds in the oven, arrange them in a single layer in a shallow baking pan in a 350°F oven for five to ten minutes, rotating them occasionally until they are very lightly browned. Sesame seeds can be toasted on the stove in an ungreased skillet just by shaking them in a hot pan for two to three minutes.

Grill or caramelize onions. Just like garlic, onions get sweeter and mellower when they are cooked. Caramelized onions are a delicious way to enhance a wide variety of dishes. Add them to bean dishes, whole grain pita sandwiches, and bean burgers. Heat a nonstick skillet until it's very hot, add sliced onions, and stir them constantly until they are tender and translucent or just lightly browned. Be careful not to burn them. Add a teaspoon or two of water if desired. After the onions are cooked, add a splash of balsamic vinegar to enhance their sweetness.

Season with spices and herbs. Season your foods with spices and fresh herbs to enhance flavor without adding fat, sugar, salt, or calories. Try fresh parsley, basil, dill, and cilantro instead of the dried versions to add fresh, distinct flavors to your dishes (the general rule of thumb is that 1 teaspoon of dried equals 1 tablespoon of fresh). The mild flavor of parsley complements many dishes. Incorporate it into your recipe or sprinkle it on top. Fresh basil is a staple of Italian cooking and shines when paired with tomatoes. Dill complements cucumbers, green beans, and other vegetable dishes. Oregano is wonderful sprinkled on salads, and cilantro adds distinctive flavor to Mexican dishes like salsa and chili as well as Asian recipes and curries. Add fresh herbs at the end of cooking for optimal flavor.

Certain herbs and spices work well together, and these combinations can be identified in many of the world's cuisines. Use Table 14 as a guide for creatively seasoning your vegetable dishes.

Use a wok without oil. A wok is like a curved frying pan, but the curved shape changes the way the food cooks. The high sides of the wok allow foods with different cooking times to be cooked together. The hardier vegetables are put in the wok first and cooked until halfway done. They are then pushed up the sides of the wok while the more tender vegetables are added. While the last ingredients cook, the first ingredients are also cooking, but at a slower rate so they don't overcook. Woks also allow you to cook greater quantities so you can have leftovers the next day. With a good nonstick skillet or wok, you can stir-fry without oil. Just heat your wok before adding the food. Add a tablespoon or two of water or low-sodium broth to prevent sticking. Stir often. Add additional water by the tablespoon as needed. Covering the pan will help the vegetables cook faster. Including ingredients with a higher water content, such as pineapple and tomatoes, will also make it easier to stir-fry without oil.

Use nutritional yeast (without folic acid). Nutritional yeast is a deactivated yeast that provides a savory, cheesy, nutty flavor. It's different from brewer's yeast, which is a product of the beer-making industry. Just a tablespoon or two of nutritional yeast can enhance soups, sauces, and salad dressings. Choose a nutritional yeast that is not fortified with folic acid. Some troubling studies have connected folic acid supplementation with breast, prostate, and colorectal cancers. (See the Appendix, where this is discussed in more detail.)

Use gourmet flavored vinegars. Vinegar is a flavor enhancer. Gourmet flavored vinegars can infuse your salads and cooked dishes with bright and bold flavors without adding oil, salt, or sugar. Stock your pantry with a variety of vinegars so that you always have the right one on hand. Try sherry vinegar, champagne vinegar, and good-quality balsamic vinegar. Experiment with a variety of fruit-flavored vinegars, such as fig, raspberry, pomegranate, orange, and pear. I'm such a fan of fruity vinegars that I've been making them available for years on my website. My favorites are still Blood Orange and Black Fig vinegars, which I use for many of my dressing recipes.

Put cinnamon on everything. You might use cinnamon in baked goods or sprinkle it on fruit or oatmeal, but it also works wonders in stews and sauces. Add a dash to your cooked leafy greens to curb bitterness, or shake a bit on your carrots or squash to enhance their natural sweetness. Look for Ceylon cinnamon, which is known as "true cinnamon." In the United States, it's more common to find cassia cinnamon, a closely related and less expensive variety; but it contains high levels of coumarin, a naturally occurring substance that has the potential to damage the liver in high doses. Ceylon cinnamon contains only traces of coumarin and has a sweeter, more delicate flavor.

7. Use beans as the major starch source.

Beans in your diet do a lot of good things for your health:

Beans lower blood pressure.[1]

Beans lower blood glucose levels.[2]

Beans lower cholesterol levels.[3]

Beans shrink your waist.[4]

Beans enhance longevity.[5]

8. Never snack on nuts; eat them with meals instead.

Eating nuts and seeds with meals enhances the absorption of phytonutrients and fat-soluble vitamins and antioxidants. But if you eat them between meals, they will spoil your appetite, and you won't be able to eat them with the vegetables at mealtime. If you're overweight, don't overeat on nuts, as they are relatively high in calories compared with other foods.

9. Buy fruit in season in bulk or right at the farm.

Having a big freezer and buying or picking fruit in the summer and freezing it in bags for the winter saves money. A big box freezer pays for itself tenfold in just a few years on all the money you save freezing fruit through the winter. When perishable food is on sale, or at a better price, you can purchase in bulk and freeze. I strongly recommend storing tomatoes and berries self-grown or purchased in season at local farms. You should also buy fresh pomegranate when in season and deseed them and store the kernels (arils) in your freezer.

10. Garden and grow some of your food.

If you have the opportunity, learn how to garden and grow more of your own food. Plant some fruit trees in your yard, such as a hazelnut or chestnut tree, and add a patch of asparagus and kale to your backyard. Making and jarring tomato sauce from tomatoes grown in your own garden is also a wonderful family activity.

Many people grow their own fig trees. What's more delicious than a fresh ripe fig? It's easy to do almost anywhere in the country. If you live in the northern part of the United States, for instance, you can grow your own fig tree in a giant outdoor pot (with a water drainage hole in the side of the pot near the bottom). Then just trim the fig tree back each November to a manageable size to be able to bring it indoors, in a shed or garage, for the winter. Six small trees can produce more than a thousand fresh figs each year.

11. Make fruit sorbets and bean treats for dinner desserts.

You can make fantastic creamy desserts merely by blending together some frozen and fresh fruits in the blender. You can make them even more diabolically delicious by adding some dried fruit that you've soaked in advance in soy, hemp, or almond milk. Use real vanilla beans (I explain how to do this in several of the recipes in Chapter 7). Try using cocoa powder or raw carob powder for a healthy chocolate

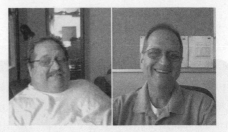

ice cream treat. It's so easy! Mix together a frozen banana, a few table-spoons of coconut flakes, two Medjool dates, and 2 teaspoons of cocoa powder—and just like that, you have a creamy chocolate ice cream.

I love a cool, tart strawberry sorbet that I make frequently for dessert. I just blend a bag of frozen strawberries with a peeled navel orange and a squeeze of lemon. You have to try it! You can even make carob or chocolate bean brownies that taste incredible and are made mostly of beans. Take a look at the dessert section starting on page 274, and you'll never miss those junk food desserts.

12. Have green smoothies for breakfast.

Many people love blending kale, lettuce, spinach, flaxseeds, or chia or hemp seeds with some fresh or frozen fruit to make a satisfying and healthy thick "blended salad" for breakfast. This is a tasty way to get your raw kale or collards in your daily diet. Remember: Raw cruciferous vegetables, blended or chewed well, give us the largest amount of isothiocyanates, which have powerful anticancer benefits. Smoothies are so easy and so quick and have made a profound difference in the health and lives of thousands of people.

Sample Menus

I have developed two weeks of sample menus for you. Week 1 requires very little work for people with little or no time to cook. It takes minimal food preparation and features a few simple easy-to-follow recipes. Week 1 makes use of store-bought salad dressings and vegetable soups. Since most salad dressings and soups contain unhealthy amounts of salt, oil, and other additives, please refer to my lists of recommended products (see Tables 15–17). Add frozen veggies (broccoli, spinach, kale, mixed vegetable blends) to the soup before you heat it up if it doesn't contain a big nutritarian serving of vegetables.

Week 2 is a more traditional nutritarian menu that includes nut/
seed-based dressings, healthful homemade vegetable bean soups, and
fruit sorbets. These menus will help you develop your nutritarian cooking skills. They feature more recipes and may require some extra time
in the kitchen, but the results are well worth it.

You may not need to make all the items on these menus each day;
adjust them to meet your own tastes and schedule. In reality, they will
probably provide more than just two meals. Leftover salad dressings
and soups are used here to make your cooking more efficient.

Remember to include different kinds of lettuce and greens, tomatoes, shredded onion, and at least one shredded raw cruciferous vegetable in your salad every day. For added veggies, choose from red and
green bell peppers, cucumbers, carrots, bean sprouts, shredded red or
green cabbage, chopped white and red onion, lightly sautéed mushrooms, lightly steamed and sliced zucchini, raw and lightly steamed
beets and carrots, snow peas, broccoli, cauliflower, and radishes. Add
different types of beans as well as some cooked vegetables for variety.

Use lemon or lime juice, flavored vinegars, herbs, and spices to
healthfully flavor your meals.

The nutritional analysis given for each day's menu is based on approximately 1,800 calories. The following meals, however, range from
1,200 to 2,400 calories, depending on your needs. If you need to lose
weight, you can modify the menus and reduce calories by omitting
dried fruits, nut butters, avocado, and bread and then reducing the
fruit a bit. If your lifestyle requires a higher caloric intake, increase
portion sizes and add more raw nuts and seeds, avocado, or unsulfured
dried fruit, such as dried figs or apricots, as well as more beans and
more intact whole grains.

Recipes for items marked with an asterisk are included in Chapter 7 of this book. And don't forget to refer to Tables 15 through 17 for
recommended purchased soups and salad dressings.

TABLE 14. FLAVORS AND FOODS OF INTERNATIONAL CUISINES

ITALIAN	THAI	MEXICAN	MOROCCAN	ASIAN	GREEK	INDIAN
Garlic	Garlic	Cumin	Garlic	Ginger	Garlic	Garlic
Onion	Shallot	Cilantro	Onions	Garlic	Mint	Ginger
Basil	Basil	Garlic	Cinnamon	Coriander	Oregano	Onion
Oregano	Lemongrass	Coriander	Ginger	Scallions	Dill	Turmeric
Thyme	Curry	Onions	Cilantro	Sesame	Chilies	Cumin
Parsley	Ginger	Chilies	Mint	Vinegar	Cinnamon	Coriander
Marjoram	Mint	Cinnamon	Saffron	Lime	Parsley	Curry blends
Rosemary	Cilantro		Cumin		Thyme	Garam masala
	Chilies		Lemon		Marjoram	
	Lime				Lemon	

PAIR WITH:	PAIR WITH:	PAIR WITH:	PAIR WITH:	PAIR WITH:	PAIR WITH:	PAIR WITH:
Tomato	Peas	Bell pepper	Eggplant	Shiitake	Arugula	Spinach
Mushrooms	Spinach	Cauliflower	Orange	Cucumber	Eggplant	Peas
Kale	Zucchini	Tomato	Tomato	Broccoli	Cucumber	Tomato
Spinach	Carrots	Corn	Carrot	Bok choy	Zucchini	Sweet potato
Bell pepper	Eggplant	Jicama	Chickpeas	Tofu		Chickpeas
Mushrooms	Broccoli	Zucchini				
White beans		Black and red beans				
		Avocado				

Week 1:
Too Busy to Cook a Nutritarian Menu

Day 1

BREAKFAST

Oatmeal with blueberries and chia seeds. *Combine ½ cup old-fashioned oats with 1 cup water or nondairy milk. Heat in microwave on high for 2 minutes, stir and microwave an additional minute. Stir in thawed frozen blueberries and chia seeds.*
One apple or banana

LUNCH

Huge salad with assorted vegetables, walnuts, and bottled low-sodium/no-oil dressing
Low-sodium purchased vegetable bean soup
One fresh or frozen fruit

DINNER

Carrot and celery sticks, cherry tomatoes, raw cauliflower, and red pepper slices with bottled low-sodium/no-oil dressing
Sunny Bean Burgers* on 100 percent whole grain pita with tomato, red onion, sautéed mushrooms, and low-sodium ketchup
Black Cherry Sorbet* or fresh or frozen fruit

NUTRITION FACTS FOR THIS MENU: CALORIES 1,785; PROTEIN 67g; CARBOHYDRATES 313g; TOTAL FAT 44g; SATURATED FAT 6g; SODIUM 637mg; FIBER 68g; BETACAROTENE 35,739mcg; VITAMIN C 468mg; CALCIUM 694mg; IRON 21mg; FOLATE 991mcg; MAGNESIUM 629mg; ZINC 13mg; SELENIUM 66mcg

PROTEIN 14.0 percent; CARBOHYDRATE 65.4 percent; TOTAL FAT 20.6 percent

---

*Asterisks indicate recipes that can be found in Chapter 7 of this book.

Day 2

> 2 pieces of fruit
> 1 ounce almonds (about ¼ cup)

> Huge salad with assorted vegetables, sliced scallions, boxed or
> canned beans, and Easy Avocado Dressing* or bottled
> low-sodium/no-oil dressing
> One slice 100 percent whole grain or sprouted grain bread (see
> Table 18)
> One fresh or frozen fruit. *Try defrosted frozen peaches sometime; just
> take them out of the freezer and place in the fridge the night before.
> They're great!*

> Salad with assorted vegetables, with leftover Easy Avocado
> Dressing* or bottled low-sodium/no-oil dressing
> Black Bean Quinoa Soup* or low-sodium purchased vegetable
> bean soup with added frozen veggies
> Banana with low-sodium, natural peanut butter or raw cashew
> butter

NUTRITION FACTS FOR THIS MENU: CALORIES 1,784; PROTEIN 74g; CARBOHY-
DRATES 254g; TOTAL FAT 69g; SATURATED FAT 10g; SODIUM 512mg; FIBER 71g;
BETA-CAROTENE 29,965mcg; VITAMIN C 466mg; CALCIUM 666mg; IRON 21mg; FO-
LATE 1,627mcg; MAGNESIUM 677mg; ZINC 12mg; SELENIUM 33mcg

PROTEIN 15.3 percent; CARBOHYDRATE 52.5 percent; TOTAL FAT 32.2 percent

Day 3

BREAKFAST

Overnight Oatmeal* with dried and fresh fruit

One navel orange

LUNCH

Huge salad with assorted vegetables, pumpkin seeds, and bottled
    low-sodium/no-oil dressing or flavored vinegar

Leftover Black Bean Quinoa Soup* or low-sodium purchased
    vegetable bean soup

One fresh or frozen fruit

DINNER

Raw vegetables with Super Simple Hummus* or bottled low-
    sodium/no-oil dressing

Sweet Potatoes Topped with Black Beans and Kale*

Fresh or frozen fruit. *Try frozen cherries; I love them left out of the
    freezer for just 15 to 20 minutes so they're still a little frozen.*

NUTRITION FACTS FOR THIS MENU: CALORIES 1,795; PROTEIN 72g; CARBOHY-
DRATES 333g; TOTAL FAT 33g; SATURATED FAT 5g; SODIUM 558mg; FIBER 72g; BETA-
CAROTENE 35,550mcg; VITAMIN C 352mg; CALCIUM 872mg; IRON 23mg; FOLATE
1,009mcg; MAGNESIUM 692mg; ZINC 11mg; SELENIUM 31mcg

PROTEIN 15.0 percent; CARBOHYDRATE 69.5 percent; TOTAL FAT 15.5 percent

Day 4

BREAKFAST

Thawed frozen blueberries or strawberries mixed with currants, crushed walnuts, and raw sunflower seeds

LUNCH

100 percent whole grain wrap or pita with mixed greens, tomato, avocado, sliced onion, and Russian Fig Dressing* or bottled low-sodium/no-oil dressing (add 2 ounces of baked chicken or turkey if desired)

One fresh fruit. *Always keep some apples on hand, because they don't get crushed when traveling with you.*

DINNER

Salad with bottled low-sodium/no-oil dressing

White Bean and Kale Soup* or low-sodium purchased vegetable bean soup with added frozen vegetables

Apple Surprise* or fresh or frozen fruit

NUTRITION FACTS FOR THIS MENU: CALORIES 1,826; PROTEIN 67g; CARBOHY-DRATES 275g; TOTAL FAT 68g; SATURATED FAT 7g; SODIUM 634mg; FIBER 61g; BETA-CAROTENE 24,348mcg; VITAMIN C 304mg; CALCIUM 771mg; IRON 22mg; FOLATE 899mcg; MAGNESIUM 608mg; ZINC 11mg; SELENIUM 65mcg

PROTEIN 13.5 percent; CARBOHYDRATE 55.6 percent; TOTAL FAT 30.9 percent

Day 5

BREAKFAST

Banana Cashew Lettuce Wrap*

LUNCH

Huge salad with assorted vegetables and bottled low-sodium/no-
oil dressing, flavored vinegar, or Orange Sesame Dressing*

Leftover White Bean and Kale Soup* or low-sodium purchased
vegetable bean soup

One fresh or frozen fruit. *Try apples or peaches dipped in Ceylon cinnamon. Ceylon cinnamon doesn't have the high levels of potentially
liver-damaging coumarin that cassia cinnamon has.*

DINNER

Raw vegetables with Super Simple Hummus* or bottled low-
sodium/no-oil dressing

Portobellos and Beans*

Fresh or frozen cooked spinach or other vegetable

One fresh or frozen fruit. *Try semi-defrosted frozen mango. It's fantastic!*

NUTRITION FACTS FOR THIS MENU: CALORIES 1,756; PROTEIN 82g; CARBOHY-
DRATES 284g; TOTAL FAT 43g; SATURATED FAT 8g; SODIUM 492mg; FIBER 66g; BETA-
CAROTENE 34,074mcg; VITAMIN C 700mg; CALCIUM 1,341mg; IRON 37mg; FOLATE
1,539mcg; MAGNESIUM 902mg; ZINC 16mg; SELENIUM 49mcg

PROTEIN 17.9 percent; CARBOHYDRATE 60.9 percent; TOTAL FAT 21.2 percent

Day 6

BREAKFAST

Eat Your Greens Fruit Smoothie*

One slice 100 percent whole grain or sprouted grain bread (see
Table 18) with raw cashew or almond butter

LUNCH

Huge salad with assorted vegetables, beans, avocado, sliced
red onion, and Walnut Vinaigrette Dressing* or bottled
low-sodium/no-oil dressing

One fresh or frozen fruit

DINNER

Salad with assorted vegetables and leftover Walnut Vinaigrette
Dressing* or bottled low-sodium/no-oil dressing

Easy Vegetable Pizza*

Blueberry Banana Cobbler* or frozen blueberries with Vanilla
Cream Topping*

NUTRITION FACTS FOR THIS MENU: CALORIES 1,798; PROTEIN 57g; CARBOHY-
DRATES 275g; TOTAL FAT 67g; SATURATED FAT 10g; SODIUM 723mg; FIBER 62g;
BETA-CAROTENE 23,839mcg; VITAMIN C 237mg; CALCIUM 803mg; IRON 21mg; FO-
LATE 1,218mcg; MAGNESIUM 656mg; ZINC 10mg; SELENIUM 71mcg

PROTEIN 11.9 percent; CARBOHYDRATE 57 percent; TOTAL FAT 31.1 percent

Day 7

Chia Breakfast Pudding* or 2 pieces of fruit. *Make or purchase raw cashew butter and mash in crushed walnuts with the back of a wooden spoon to make cashew-walnut spread to use on fruit or fennel and celery sticks.*

Huge salad with assorted vegetables, almonds or walnuts, and Russian Fig Dressing* or bottled low-sodium/no-oil dressing or flavored vinegar
Mexican Lentils* or low-sodium purchased vegetable bean soup
Fresh or frozen fruit

Raw veggies with Fresh Tomato Salsa* or bottled low-sodium salsa
Black Bean and Turkey Burgers* (recipe includes vegan option) on whole grain pita with avocado, lettuce, and tomato
Fresh or frozen steamed broccoli. *Rub raw broccoli lightly with a splash of olive oil and steam with sliced garlic.*
Fresh fruit

NUTRITION FACTS FOR THIS MENU: CALORIES 1,855; PROTEIN 76g; CARBOHY-DRATES 275g; TOTAL FAT 66g; SATURATED FAT 8g; SODIUM 823mg; FIBER 93g; BETA-CAROTENE 35,678mcg; VITAMIN C 497mg; CALCIUM 927mg; IRON 25mg; FOLATE 1,969mcg; MAGNESIUM 697mg; ZINC 16mg; SELENIUM 75mcg

PROTEIN 15.1 percent; CARBOHYDRATE 55.2 percent; TOTAL FAT 29.7 percent

Week 2:
Nutritarian Menus with a Bit More Cooking

Day 1

BREAKFAST

Kale Power Blended Salad*

Splurge with a small box of fresh raspberries or cup of defrosted frozen berries.

LUNCH

Huge salad with assorted vegetables and bottled low-sodium/ no-oil dressing or flavored vinegar

One slice 100 percent whole grain or sprouted grain bread (see Table 18), with mashed avocado and pan-grilled onion slices

Fresh or frozen fruit

DINNER

Creamy Cabbage Soup*

Chopped kale tossed with Orange Sesame Dressing* served over black bean pasta

Chunky Blueberry Walnut Sorbet* or fresh fruit

NUTRITION FACTS FOR THIS MENU: CALORIES 1,748; PROTEIN 61g; CARBOHY-DRATES 296g; TOTAL FAT 54g; SATURATED FAT 8g; SODIUM 677mg; FIBER 68g; BETA-CAROTENE 49,521mcg; VITAMIN C 794mg; CALCIUM 1,156mg; IRON 23mg; FOLATE 963mcg; MAGNESIUM 665mg; ZINC 11mg; SELENIUM 39mcg

PROTEIN 12.7 percent; CARBOHYDRATE 61.8 percent; TOTAL FAT 25.5 percent

Day 2

BREAKFAST

> Chia Breakfast Pudding*
>
> 1 ounce walnuts (about ¼ cup)

LUNCH

> Huge salad with assorted vegetables, sliced red onion, and Creamy
>   Almond Vinaigrette Dressing* or bottled low-sodium/no-oil
>   dressing or flavored vinegar
> Leftover Creamy Cabbage Soup*
> Sliced apple dipped in Ceylon cinnamon

DINNER

> Flax and Sesame Crackers* with Mediterranean Tomato Spread*
> Ratatouille over Spaghetti Squash*
> Grilled asparagus
> Fresh or frozen fruit

NUTRITION FACTS FOR THIS MENU: CALORIES 1,765; PROTEIN 70g; CARBOHY-
DRATES 247g; TOTAL FAT 71g; SATURATED FAT 8g; SODIUM 612mg; FIBER 64g; BETA-
CAROTENE 40,466mcg; VITAMIN C 447mg; CALCIUM 1,026mg; IRON 27mg; FOLATE
953mcg; MAGNESIUM 719mg; ZINC 12mg; SELENIUM 43mcg

PROTEIN 14.7 percent; CARBOHYDRATE 51.8 percent; TOTAL FAT 33.5 percent

Day 3

BREAKFAST

Apple Pie Oatmeal*

Hemp Almond Milk* (1 glass)

LUNCH

Kale and Quinoa Salad with Blueberries and Mangoes*

Tofu Fingers Marinara*

DINNER

Salad with assorted vegetables and Southwest Ranch Dressing*

In-a-Hurry Anticancer Soup*

Cocoa Ice Bean* or fresh or frozen fruit

NUTRITION FACTS FOR THIS MENU: CALORIES 1,776; PROTEIN 70g; CARBOHY-DRATES 235g; TOTAL FAT 77g; SATURATED FAT 10g; SODIUM 448mg; FIBER 46g; BETA-CAROTENE 43,242mcg; VITAMIN C 323mg; CALCIUM 1,178mg; IRON 23mg; FOLATE 871mcg; MAGNESIUM 802mg; ZINC 13mg; SELENIUM 46mcg

PROTEIN 14.7 percent; CARBOHYDRATE 50.1 percent; TOTAL FAT 35.2 percent

Day 4

BREAKFAST

Mixed fruit plate topped with chia seeds

One slice 100 percent whole grain or sprouted grain bread
(see Table 18) with *trans* fat–free spread

LUNCH

Huge salad with assorted vegetables and avocado with leftover
Southwest Ranch Dressing*

Leftover In-a-Hurry Anticancer Soup* or low-sodium purchased
vegetable bean soup

Fresh fruit

DINNER

Raw broccoli with Fresh Tomato Salsa.* *If you like your salsa hot and
spicy, add some of the seeds from the jalapeños.*

Vegetable Chickpea Loaf*

California Creamed Kale*

Oatmeal Raisin Cookies Filled with Blueberry Jam*

NUTRITION FACTS FOR THIS MENU: CALORIES 1,794; PROTEIN 60g; CARBOHY-
DRATES 277g; TOTAL FAT 66g; SATURATED FAT 11g; SODIUM 784mg; FIBER 53g;
BETA-CAROTENE 51,682mcg; VITAMIN C 620mg; CALCIUM 895mg; IRON 21mg; FO-
LATE 877mcg; MAGNESIUM 668mg; ZINC 11mg; SELENIUM 69mcg

PROTEIN 12.3 percent; CARBOHYDRATE 57.2 percent; TOTAL FAT 30.5 percent

Day 5

BREAKFAST

> Veggie Scramble*
>
> Cinnamon Currant Muffin*

LUNCH

> Whole grain wrap or pita with mixed greens, tomato, and
>   Super Simple Hummus*
>
> Kale Chips*
>
> One fresh or frozen fruit

DINNER

> Salad with assorted vegetables, sliced red onion, and Russian
>   Fig Dressing*
>
> Greens, Beans, and Mushroom Stew*
>
> Crispy Mushroom Fries* or grilled corn on the cob
>
> Mixed fresh or frozen berries

NUTRITION FACTS FOR THIS MENU: CALORIES 1,728; PROTEIN 80g; CARBOHY-
DRATES 277g; TOTAL FAT 47g; SATURATED FAT 9g; SODIUM 790mg; FIBER 74g; BETA-
CAROTENE 31,844mcg; VITAMIN C 344mg; CALCIUM 819mg; IRON 25mg; FOLATE
1,346mcg; MAGNESIUM 641mg; ZINC 14mg; SELENIUM 87mcg

PROTEIN 17.2 percent; CARBOHYDRATE 59.9 percent; TOTAL FAT 32.9 percent

Day 6

BREAKFAST

Overnight Oatmeal*

LUNCH

Huge salad with assorted vegetables and Pistachio Mint Dressing*
or no-oil/low-sodium salad dressing
Leftover Greens, Beans, and Mushroom Stew*
One fresh or frozen fruit

DINNER

Carrots, red pepper, and Belgium endive with Avocado Pumpkin
Seed Salsa*
White Bean, Wild Rice, and Almond Burgers* or Meat-Lover's
Beef, Bean, and Mushroom Burgers* on a whole grain pita with
sautéed mushrooms, lettuce, and tomato
Sweet and Smoky Baked Beans*
Fresh or frozen fruit

NUTRITION FACTS FOR THIS MENU (White Bean, Wild Rice, and Almond Burger used
for calculations): CALORIES 1,818; PROTEIN 82g; CARBOHYDRATES 303g; TOTAL FAT
44g; SATURATED FAT 6g; SODIUM 741mg; FIBER 80g; BETA-CAROTENE 20,831mcg;
VITAMIN C 455mg; CALCIUM 662mg; IRON 26mg; FOLATE 1,237mcg; MAGNESIUM
698mg; ZINC 14mg; SELENIUM 54mcg

PROTEIN 16.9 percent; CARBOHYDRATE 62.6 percent; TOTAL FAT 20.5 percent

Day 7

BREAKFAST

Mixed Berries and Greens Smoothie*

1 ounce raw almonds (about ¼ cup)

LUNCH

Baja Mango Black Bean Lettuce Wrap*

Flax and Sesame Crackers* with leftover Avocado Pumpkin
    Seed Salsa*

Fresh or frozen fruit

DINNER

Salad with assorted vegetables and leftover Pistachio Mint Dressing*

Bean Pasta with Cauliflower in a Garlicky Walnut Sauce*

Vanilla Coconut Nice Cream* with fresh or frozen berries

NUTRITION FACTS FOR THIS MENU: CALORIES 1,759; PROTEIN 62g; CARBOHY-
DRATES 204g; TOTAL FAT 92g; SATURATED FAT 20g; SODIUM 259mg; FIBER 61g;
BETA-CAROTENE 10,724mcg; VITAMIN C 304mg; CALCIUM 789mg; IRON 19mg; FO-
LATE 937mcg; MAGNESIUM 774mg; ZINC 11mg; SELENIUM 32mcg

PROTEIN 13.3 percent; CARBOHYDRATE 43.1 percent; TOTAL FAT 43.6 percent

Soup and Salad Dressing
Recommendations

In Tables 15, 16, and 17 I make some recommendations for store-bought soups and salad dressings. Some contain sweeteners, preservatives, or other ingredients that I wouldn't use in my own products, but they are better choices than others in their categories because they are lower in sodium and calories than the majority of comparable products.

A natural, unprocessed, plant-based diet provides 500 to 750 milligrams of sodium per day. I recommend that women stay under 900 milligrams of sodium per day and men under 1,200 milligrams per day. Most prepared foods contain very high levels of sodium, so when you use prepared products, choose carefully.

Table 15 shows soups that contain less than 150 milligrams of sodium per cup and use BPA-free packaging; Table 16 lists soups that are a little higher in sodium. I recommend the lower sodium ones for regular use. The higher sodium soups are suitable for occasional use or 1 cup a day, as long as you're not eating any other foods with added sodium. Keep in mind that you're likely to consume more than 1 cup, which will add additional sodium.

Broths and creamy soups that can be used as convenient bases are also included in the tables. Add your own cooked beans and fresh or frozen vegetables to create a more complete nutrient-dense meal.

Soups packaged in cartons are generally better choices than soups in cans. As I've said, the lining of many metal cans contains BPA, a chemical that exhibits hormone-disrupting properties. Disruption of hormone levels due to BPA has been linked to breast cancer, prostate cancer, cardiovascular disease, diabetes, infertility, birth defects, miscarriages, developmental disorders in girls, premature puberty in young girls, severe attention deficit disorder, cognitive and brain development problems, deformations of the body, sexual development problems, and feminizing of males or masculine effects on females. Research has also indicated that BPA disturbs body weight regulation and promotes obesity and insulin resistance.[6] Some companies are now in the process of switching to cans that do not contain BPA. The products I list in Tables 15 and 16 are packaged in cartons or in cans claimed to be BPA-free.

Product information may change, so always check labels and nutrition facts before you buy. If I do not list a product as BPA-free here, it does not mean that a company's products contain it. I advise you to check with the manufacturer because some companies are in the process of removing it from their packaging.

People sometimes say ... I would rather enjoy my life more eating unhealthfully, even if I die younger. But eating unhealthfully does not lead to more enjoyment of life; that is a fallacy. There is a learning curve and your taste can get stronger as you get healthier. Plus, once people become seriously ill, they almost always want to take that back.

Think of the you twenty years from now. What would the future you advise you to do today?

Don't worry if you don't feel well at first when you change your diet. It is normal to feel poorly for a few weeks. It is also normal to miss the foods you are addicted to. It may take effort at first, but the benefits you can get from superior nutrition are priceless. With time, your taste preferences change and you actually can prefer the flavor of foods that protect your precious health. It can take a few months, but you not only are what you eat, but you prefer to eat what you eat. The more you eat healthy foods, the more you want to eat healthy foods.

Since eating healthfully is just as pleasurable (eventually) as eating to create disease, it becomes crazy to earn a heart attack, stroke, or dementia with conventional food. Nutritarians are normal; everyone else is insane.

TABLE 15. BPA-FREE SOUPS (less than 150 mg sodium/cup): RECOMMENDED

PRODUCT	SODIUM (mg/cup)	COMMENTS
Dr. Fuhrman's VitaBean	135	Carton
Dr. Fuhrman's Moroccan Chickpea	95	Carton
Dr. Fuhrman's Supreme Greens	120	Carton
Pacific Foods Low Sodium Vegetable Broth	135	Broth/stock—use as a base; carton
Pacific Foods Simply Stock— Vegetable	65	Broth/stock—use as a base; carton
Imagine Foods Low Sodium Vegetable Broth	140	Broth/stock—use as a base; contains oil; carton
Imagine Foods Low Sodium No-Chicken Broth	140	Broth/stock—use as a base; contains oil; carton
Imagine Foods Light Sodium Sweet Potato	140	Creamy—use as a base; contains white potatoes, organic rice syrup, and oil; carton
Trader Joe's Low Sodium Butternut Squash	90	Creamy—use as a base; contains white potatoes and evaporated cane sugar; carton
Trader Joe's Low Sodium Vegetable Broth	140	Broth/stock—use as a base; contains olive oil; carton
Health Valley No Salt Added Organic Vegetable	50	Vitamin A palmitate added; contains evaporated cane juice and oil; BPA-free can
Health Valley No Salt Added Lentil	30	Vitamin A palmitate added; contains evaporated cane juice and oil; BPA-free can

TABLE 17. CANNED SOUPS (less than 300 mg sodium/cup):
USE ONLY RARELY (BPA in can lining)

PRODUCT	SODIUM (mg/cup)	COMMENTS
Health Valley No Salt Added Organic Vegetable	50	Vitamin A palmitate added; contains evaporated cane juice and oil
Health Valley No Salt Added Lentil	30	Vitamin A palmitate added; contains evaporated cane juice and oil
Health Valley No Salt Added Minestrone	50	Vitamin A palmitate added; contains evaporated cane juice and oil
Health Valley No Salt Added Black Bean	30	Contains cane juice and oil
Health Valley No Salt Added Mushroom Barley	60	Vitamin A palmitate added; contains cane juice and oil
Pritikin Chunky Vegetable Low Sodium	80	Contains sugar and oil
Trader Joe's Low Sodium Minestrone	140	Contains pasta, egg whites, sugar, and oil

Table 17 lists salad dressings that contain no more than 150 milligrams of sodium per serving. They don't contain refined oils, including olive oil, which are high in calories yet provide little nutritional value.

Instead of low-nutrient, refined oils, I use nuts, seeds, and avocados as the fat sources in my dressings. They are ideal in salad dressings because they enhance the absorption of nutrients from the vegetables in the salad. We need to eat healthful fats the way nature intended, in whole natural foods. If you use an oil-based dressing or olive oil occasionally, limit yourself to 1 tablespoon or mix with a more favorable dressing.

TABLE 17. NO-OIL SALAD DRESSINGS (150 mg sodium or less / 2 tablespoons): RECOMMENDED

PRODUCT	SODIUM mg/2 tbl	CALORIES/ 2 tbl	COMMENTS
Dr. Fuhrman's Sesame Ginger	5	60	
Dr. Fuhrman's Almond Balsamic	0	45	
Dr. Fuhrman's Tuscan Herb	0	35	
Dr. Fuhrman's Blueberry Pom	0	45	
Dr. Fuhrman's Walnut Vinaigrette	0	70	
Dr. Fuhrman's Orange Cashew	0	50	
Whole Foods Health Starts Here Sesame Ginger	115	70	
Whole Foods Health Starts Here Balsamic Dressing	40	30	
Whole Foods Health Starts Here Tomato Basil	80	20	
Whole Foods Health Starts Here Pomegranate Vinaigrette	70	35	
Whole Foods Health Starts Here Carrot Ginger	90	40	

Whole Foods Health Starts Here Avocado Vinaigrette	45	25	
Whole Foods Health Starts Here Vegan Caesar	20	20	
Annie's Naturals Fat-Free Raspberry Balsamic Vinaigrette	10	30	Contains cane sugar
Annie's Naturals Fat-Free Mango Vinaigrette	5	20	Contains cane sugar
Maple Grove Farms Balsamic Vinaigrette	120	15	Contains sugar
Maple Grove Farms Lime Basil	150	25	Contains sugar
Maple Grove Farms Vidalia Onion	150	20	Contains sugar
Kozlowski Farms Raspberry Poppy	90	25	Contains cane sugar
Kozlowski Farms Fat Free Honey Mustard	120	35	Contains cane sugar
Consorzio Fat Free Raspberry & Balsamic	10	15	Contains sugar

Dr. Fuhrman Foods

Some people may object to my promoting my own products here. A few have even voiced their concern that my message is driven by commerce, which trumps my scientific message and integrity. I want to address that up front and state that offering products that allow people to maintain their commitment to healthy eating is consistent with my mission of enabling people to transform their lives and reverse and restore their good health and prevent disease in their future.

I was fortunate to be able to respond to a critical need and numerous public requests. When I started developing my products, there were simply no options for busy people who wanted to commit to a nutritarian lifestyle but who had no time to prepare healthy foods from scratch. There weren't any no-salt-added prepared soups without BPA in the marketplace; there were no nut/seed-based salad dressings without salt and oil. Hundreds of people asked me to develop "medical foods" that can be used by heart patients and diabetics and health seekers so that these miraculous results of healing and recovery are easier, and in some cases even possible, to incorporate in their lives. My support team and I developed the Dr. Fuhrman products, and we have been rewarded with transformational success stories and letters of gratitude.

My products meet a need that isn't met elsewhere. They are made in relatively small batches, with high-quality ingredients and therefore are relatively expensive to manufacture. I also recommend many other products that come close to meeting specific health criteria. I hope that other companies will develop and make available more healthful commercial food options, and I expect this to happen as this nutritarian food message becomes more mainstream. Making foods from scratch in your own kitchen is certainly preferable—it's less expensive and can be even tastier when you use high-quality fresh ingredients. Purchasing prepared foods is only an option when preparing everything fresh yourself isn't possible and otherwise would make nutritarian eating too difficult for you to maintain.

Importantly, my product sales enable support for the Nutritional Research Foundation, a 501c3 foundation that initiates and funds the development of nutritional research. Purchases enable the continuation of much-needed research in this field of nutritional medicine, which is aimed at changing the face of healthcare worldwide. This research is essential to saving ourselves from the onslaught of pharmacological drugs and invasive medical procedures that ignore causation. So these purchases are also supporting a good cause.

In Their Own Words

Rod's doctor concluded that genetics predetermined Rod's health and that medication was the only solution. Rod refused to accept that and found that a nutritarian approach was his answer.

WEIGHT BEFORE: 215 pounds

WEIGHT AFTER: 145 pounds

TOTAL CHOLESTEROL BEFORE: 231

TOTAL CHOLESTEROL AFTER: 127

I had just received the results of my annual physical. For the fourth straight year, my total cholesterol was over 215; this year it was 231. The doctor called me and wanted me to start taking a statin drug. Why, I wondered, did I have to take medicine to reduce my cholesterol?

One December evening I received an e-mail from a friend. She had read Dr. Fuhrman's *Eat for Health,* had been following the nutritarian diet style for five months, and had seen her cholesterol level drop drastically. That's when I realized I had found the answer to my dilemma.

After three days of exercise and eating according to Dr. Fuhrman's advice, I lost 6 pounds! As I continued to eat green vegetables, fruits, beans, and a few nuts, I started to feel better. My cravings for processed foods and bad carbohydrates began to fade away. My energy level improved, and I was inspired to eat the foods that fueled my body.

About eight weeks later, I had my cholesterol rechecked. My total cholesterol had dropped from 231 to 127. My HDL went from 35 to 34. My LDL dropped from 168 to 82, and my triglycerides dropped from 142 to 56. Doctors told me I was just fighting genetics, yet this program proved otherwise.

Dr. Fuhrman's approach is successful because it focuses on what you *can* eat. You don't have to count points or measure out food—you just have to eat the *right* foods. I've tried many diets, but they weren't sustainable. Dr. Fuhrman's approach teaches you how to eat for a lifetime! My "new" favorite foods are my famous vegetable soup, smoothies, and best of all, my evening bowl of fresh pineapple with frozen blueberries and blackberries.

This diet style has brought me other life benefits as well: I no longer need a daily nap, for instance, and I run 7.5 miles a day. A nutritarian diet has also eliminated my cravings for toxic foods. And another added benefit: Old friends and relatives can't believe how good I look!

Your Efforts to Eat Right Are Wise and Well Spent

More medical care doesn't result in a longer-lived and healthier population. A healthy lifestyle and diet style are the only significant predictors of a healthy and long life. You can't rely on luck to get rich; nor can you rely on luck, or even genetics, to achieve excellent health. Longevity must be earned. There's no better investment of your time, attention, and money to take the best possible care of your health. That means seeking out high-quality natural foods and preparing the best meals possible for you and your family.

You really are what you eat, or said another way: You become what you once ate. When you are exposed through life to negative elements, toxins, and disease-promoting foods, they cumulatively take their toll. A healthy brain is our greatest gift; we must remember that our physical and emotional health are intertwined. Our intelligence and memory, our mood and happiness, depend on our proper food choices.

Though people love to believe that moderation in harmful substances and unhealthy foods won't hurt them, this simply is not true. Certainly our genetic makeup determines varying sensitivities to a toxic diet, but our lives are finite, and the more our bodies are stressed dealing with poor food choices, the more we squander our ultimate health and life potential. Eating unhealthfully isn't free. Ultimately, we must all pay a price.

CHAPTER SEVEN

Recipes

Juices and Smoothies

Breakfast Options

Salad Dressings, Dips, and Spreads

Salads

Soups

Main Dishes and Vegetable Side Dishes

Burgers, Pizza, and Fast Food

Desserts

JUICES AND SMOOTHIES

Hemp Almond Milk

Serves: 6

> 1 cup hulled hemp seeds
> 1 cup raw almonds, soaked 6–8 hours
> 2 Medjool or 4 Deglet Noor dates, pitted
> 4 cups water
> ½ vanilla bean, split lengthwise, or ½ teaspoon alcohol-free
>   vanilla extract

Place all ingredients in a high-powered blender. If using a vanilla bean, scrape interior pulp and seeds from pod with a dull knife and add to the blender; discard pod. Blend until smooth. If desired, strain through a nut milk bag or fine mesh strainer.

PER SERVING: CALORIES 263; PROTEIN 9g; CARBOHYDRATES 16g; TOTAL FAT 20.1g; SATURATED FAT 1.6g; SODIUM 17mg; FIBER 8.1g; BETA-CAROTENE 8mcg; CALCIUM 110mg; IRON 2mg; FOLATE 25mcg; MAGNESIUM 146mg; ZINC 1.6mg; SELENIUM 5.4mcg

Super Veggie Juice

Serves: 1

> 3 cups kale
> 1 cup broccoli
> 1 cucumber
> 2 carrots
> 1 apple
> ½-inch piece of ginger root
> ½ lemon, peeled

Run all ingredients through a juicer.

PER SERVING: CALORIES 155; PROTEIN 9g; CARBOHYDRATES 36g; TOTAL FAT 1.3g; SATURATED FAT 0.2g; SODIUM 104mg; FIBER 2g; BETA-CAROTENE 14,577mcg; VITMIN C 180mg; CALCIUM 212mg; IRON 2.7mg; FOLATE 85mcg; MAGNESIUM 77mg; ZINC 1.1mg; SELENIUM 2.6mcg

Eat Your Greens Fruit Smoothie

Serves: 2

> 5 ounces baby kale and baby spinach
> 1 banana
> 1 cup frozen or fresh blueberries
> ½ cup unsweetened soy, hemp, or almond milk
> ½ cup pomegranate juice or other unsweetened fruit juice
> 1 tablespoon ground flaxseeds

Blend all ingredients in a high-powered blender until smooth and creamy.

PER SERVING: CALORIES 201; PROTEIN 6g; CARBOHYDRATES 39g; TOTAL FAT 3.6g; SATURATED FAT 0.4g; SODIUM 94mg; FIBER 6.9g; BETA-CAROTENE 4,245mcg; VITAMIN C 27mg; CALCIUM 111mg; IRON 3.1mg; FOLATE 167mcg; MAGNESIUM 105mg; ZINC 0.9mg; SELENIUM 5.1mcg

Kale Power Blended Salad

Serves: 2

> 2 ounces kale
> 3 ounces romaine lettuce
> 1 banana
> ½ avocado
> 2 Medjool or 4 Deglet Noor dates, pitted

In a food processor or high-powered blender, blend all ingredients well until a smooth pudding-like consistency.

PER SERVING: CALORIES 211; PROTEIN 3g; CARBOHYDRATES 39g; TOTAL FAT 7g; SATURATED FAT 1g; SODIUM 32mg; FIBER 8g; BETA-CAROTENE 3,139mcg; VITAMIN C 27mg; CALCIUM 68mg; IRON 1.9mg; FOLATE 166mcg; MAGNESIUM 70mg; ZINC 1mg; SELENIUM 1.2mcg

Mixed Berries and Greens Smoothie

Serves: 2

1 cup pomegranate juice
¼ cup unsweetened soy, hemp, or almond milk
2 cups frozen mixed berries
1 cup romaine lettuce
1 cup watercress
½ banana
2 tablespoons ground chia seeds

Blend ingredients in a high-powered blender until smooth and creamy.

PER SERVING: CALORIES 223; PROTEIN 4g; CARBOHYDRATES 45g; TOTAL FAT 3.9g; SATURATED FAT 0.4g; SODIUM 36mg; FIBER 6.9g; BETA-CAROTENE 1,613mcg; VITAMIN C 78mg; CALCIUM 84mg; IRON 2.2mg; FOLATE 82mcg; MAGNESIUM 67mg; ZINC 0.8mg; SELENIUM 4.8mcg

BREAKFAST OPTIONS

Apple Pie Oatmeal
Serves: 2

½ cup old-fashioned oats
1 cup water
2 apples, peeled, cored, and diced
¼ teaspoon ground Ceylon cinnamon (see Note)
2 pitted dates, finely chopped
2 tablespoons chopped walnuts

Place oats and water in small pot and bring to a gentle boil. Reduce heat to low and simmer for 5 minutes. Stir in apples, ground cinnamon, and chopped dates. Add additional water if desired to adjust consistency. When oatmeal and apples are heated through, remove from heat and stir in walnuts.

Note: Ceylon cinnamon is known as "true cinnamon." What is commonly found in the United States is cassia cinnamon, a closely related and less expensive variety. Ceylon cinnamon is preferable because the cassia variety contains high levels of coumarin, a naturally occurring substance that has the potential to damage the liver in high doses. The Ceylon variety contains only traces of coumarin.

PER SERVING: CALORIES 220; PROTEIN 7g; CARBOHYDRATES 40g; TOTAL FAT 6.5g; SATURATED FAT 0.7g; SODIUM 5mg; FIBER 6.5g; BETA-CAROTENE 39mcg; VITAMIN C 6mg; CALCIUM 22mg; IRON 1.3mg; FOLATE 21mcg; MAGNESIUM 77mg; ZINC 1.0mg; SELENIUM 7.4mcg

Banana Cashew Lettuce Wrap

Serves: 2

> ¼ cup raw cashew butter
> 12 romaine lettuce leaves
> 2 bananas, thinly sliced

Spread about 1 teaspoon cashew butter on each lettuce leaf. Place a few banana slices on the cashew butter and roll up like a burrito.

PER SERVING: CALORIES 312; PROTEIN 8g; CARBOHYDRATES 39g; TOTAL FAT 16.5g; SATURATED FAT 3.3g; SODIUM 15mg; FIBER 6.1g; BETA-CAROTENE 3,933mcg; VITA-MIN C 37mg; CALCIUM 57mg; IRON 3mg; FOLATE 198mcg; MAGNESIUM 130mg; ZINC 2.1mg; SELENIUM 5.3mcg

Chia Breakfast Pudding

Serves: 2

> 1 cup unsweetened vanilla soy, hemp, or almond milk
> ¼ cup whole chia seeds
> ¼ cup rolled oats
> ½ vanilla bean, split lengthwise, or ½ teaspoon alcohol-free vanilla extract
> 2 tablespoons raisins
> ¼ cup blueberries
> ½ sliced banana

In a bowl, mix together all ingredients except blueberries and banana. If using a vanilla bean, scrape pulp and seeds from pod with a dull knife and add them to mixture along with the pod. Let sit for 10 minutes. (For an on-the-run breakfast, make the night before and store in the refrigerator.) Remove vanilla pod, stir in blueberries and banana. Add additional nondairy milk if desired to adjust consistency.

PER SERVING: CALORIES 265; PROTEIN 13g; CARBOHYDRATES 38g; TOTAL FAT 9.4g; SATURATED FAT 1.1g; SODIUM 71mg; FIBER 11.6g; BETA-CAROTENE 454mcg; VITA-MIN C 8mg; CALCIUM 179mg; IRON 4.1mg; FOLATE 53mcg; MAGNESIUM 84mg; ZINC 1.6mg; SELENIUM 9.5mcg

Cinnamon Currant Muffins

Serves: 12

1 cup whole wheat flour
½ cup oat flour (see Note)
1 teaspoon baking powder
1 teaspoon baking soda
3 tablespoons ground flaxseeds
1½ cups cooked white beans, or 1 (15-ounce) can no-salt-added
    or low-sodium white beans, drained
3 ripe bananas, divided
1 cup dates, pitted (preferably Medjool dates)
2 tablespoons alcohol-free vanilla extract
1½ tablespoons Ceylon cinnamon
1 tablespoon nutmeg
¾ cup dried currants

Preheat oven to 350°F. In a large bowl, sift together the whole wheat flour, oat flour, baking powder, and baking soda. In a small bowl, combine the ground flaxseeds with ½ cup water, stir, and let sit for a few minutes.

In a high-powered blender or food processor, blend beans, two of the bananas, dates, vanilla, cinnamon, nutmeg, and flaxseed/water gel. Stir blended mixture into the flour mixture. Cut remaining banana in large chunks and stir in along with currants.

Line muffin tray with paper muffin cups or spray with cooking spray. Fill each cup ¾ full. Bake for about 25 minutes or until a toothpick inserted in the center comes out clean.

Note: You can purchase oat flour in most large supermarkets or health food stores, or make it yourself by processing old-fashioned oats in a food processor or blender until ground.

PER SERVING: CALORIES 195; PROTEIN 5g; CARBOHYDRATES 42g; TOTAL FAT 1.9g; SATURATED FAT 0.4g; SODIUM 109mg; FIBER 7.6g; BETA-CAROTENE 13mcg; VITA-MIN C 3mg; CALCIUM 72mg; IRON 2.2mg; FOLATE 47mcg; MAGNESIUM 56mg; ZINC 0.8mg; SELENIUM 8.6mcg

Orange Goji Bars

Serves: 15

> 1½ cups old-fashioned oats
> 1 cup chopped walnuts
> ½ cup dates, pitted
> 1 cup unsulfured dried apricots
> 1 cup Goji berries (see Note)
> 2 tablespoons unhulled sesame seeds
> 2 tablespoons ground chia seeds
> 2 teaspoons dried organic orange zest

In a food processor, process oats until finely chopped, then add walnuts and process until chopped but not a powder. Remove to a mixing bowl.

Place dates, apricots, Goji berries, and 1 tablespoon water in food processor. Process until a large ball begins to form. Turn into mixing bowl and add sesame seeds, chia seeds, and orange zest along with the oat mixture and knead by hand until thoroughly combined. Press into an 8-by-11½-inch baking pan and cut into 15 bars.

Note: Goji berries are burnt-red in color and about the size of a raisin. They taste like a cross between a raisin, a cranberry, and a cherry. They are slightly sweet and tart. You can also use unsulfured, unsweetened dried blueberries or cherries.

PER SERVING: CALORIES 155; PROTEIN 4g; CARBOHYDRATES 22g; TOTAL FAT 6.8g; SATURATED FAT 0.7g; SODIUM 25mg; FIBER 3.5g; BETA-CAROTENE 191mcg; VITA-MIN C 20mg; CALCIUM 35mg; IRON 2.1mg; FOLATE 16mcg; MAGNESIUM 47mg; ZINC 0.7mg; SELENIUM 3.5mcg

Overnight Oatmeal

Serves: 3

> ¼ cup raisins and/or other chopped dried fruits
> 1 cup old-fashioned rolled oats
> 2 cups unsweetened soy, hemp, or almond milk
> 3 cups fresh chopped fruit or frozen mixed berries

Place the dried fruit, oats, and nondairy milk in a container. Cover and refrigerate overnight to soften. In the morning, mix with fresh chopped fruit or defrosted frozen berries. You can also add the frozen berries to the mixture the night before so you don't have to defrost them in the morning.

PER SERVING: CALORIES 298; PROTEIN 11g; CARBOHYDRATES 54g; TOTAL FAT 6.1g; SATURATED FAT 0.7g; SODIUM 91mg; FIBER 9.4g; BETA-CAROTENE 631mcg; VITAMIN C 4mg; CALCIUM 79mg; IRON 3.5mg; FOLATE 48mcg; MAGNESIUM 124mg; ZINC 1.7mg; SELENIUM 17mcg

Veggie Scramble

Serves: 2

3 cups baby spinach or baby kale
1 cup chopped onion
1 cup chopped green pepper
1 cup diced tomatoes
8 ounces (½ block) firm tofu (or 3 eggs—see Note)
1 tablespoon Dr. Fuhrman's VegiZest,* Mrs. Dash seasoning
   blend, or no-salt Spike, to taste

Water-sauté spinach or kale, onions, peppers, and tomatoes until tender. Wrap the tofu in a towel and squeeze out as much water as you can, then crumble it over the vegetable mixture and cook until tofu is lightly browned. Add seasoning.

Note: You can make this recipe with eggs instead of tofu. Blend 3 eggs with ¼ cup nondairy milk, pour over the vegetable mixture, and cook until eggs are done. It's also excellent with 2 eggs and the tofu crumbled in, in which case it can serve 3–4 people.

*A Dr. Fuhrman no-salt seasoning and green food supplement mix.

PER SERVING: CALORIES 199; PROTEIN 14g; CARBOHYDRATES 19g; TOTAL FAT 8.7g; SATURATED FAT 2.5g; SODIUM 157mg; FIBER 4.9g; BETA-CAROTENE 2,695mcg; VITAMIN C 101mg; CALCIUM 119mg; IRON 3.6mg; FOLATE 160mcg; MAGNESIUM 70mg; ZINC 1.4mg; SELENIUM 25mcg

SALAD DRESSINGS, DIPS, AND SPREADS

Creamy Almond Vinaigrette Dressing
Serves: 6

1 cup unsweetened soy, hemp, or almond milk
1 cup raw almonds or ½ cup raw almond butter
¼ cup balsamic vinegar
2 tablespoons fresh lemon juice
¼ cup raisins
2 teaspoons Dijon mustard
1 clove garlic

Blend all ingredients in a high-powered blender until creamy and smooth.

PER SERVING: CALORIES 184; PROTEIN 5g; CARBOHYDRATES 14g; TOTAL FAT 13.1g; SATURATED FAT 1.3g; SODIUM 68mg; FIBER 1.5g; BETA-CAROTENE 147mcg; VITAMIN C 3mg; CALCIUM 79mg; IRON 1.4mg; FOLATE 21mcg; MAGNESIUM 77mg; ZINC 0.8mg; SELENIUM 2mcg

Easy Avocado Dressing
Serves: 4

  2 avocados
  1 lime, juiced
  1 clove garlic, minced
  ¼ cup minced onion
  2 tablespoons nutritional yeast
  ⅛ teaspoon cayenne pepper or more to taste
  ¼ cup water

Place all ingredients in a high-powered blender or food processor and puree until smooth. Add additional water if needed to adjust consistency.

PER SERVING: CALORIES 172; PROTEIN 4g; CARBOHYDRATES 13g; TOTAL FAT 13.7g; SATURATED FAT 1.9g; SODIUM 11mg; FIBER 7.8g; BETA-CAROTENE 72mcg; VITAMIN C 14mg; CALCIUM 25mg; IRON 1.7mg; FOLATE 221mcg; MAGNESIUM 33mg; ZINC 1mg; SELENIUM 2mcg

Orange Sesame Dressing

Serves: 3

> 3 tablespoons unhulled sesame seeds, divided
> ¼ cup raw cashew nuts, or 2 tablespoons raw cashew butter
> 2 oranges, peeled
> 2 tablespoons Dr. Fuhrman's Blood Orange* or Riesling Reserve*
>   Vinegar or white wine vinegar
> Orange juice, if needed to adjust consistency

Toast the sesame seeds in a dry skillet over medium high heat for 3 minutes, mixing with a wooden spoon and shaking the pan frequently. In a high-powered blender, combine 2 tablespoons of the sesame seeds and the cashews, oranges, and vinegar. If needed, add orange juice to adjust consistency. Sprinkle remaining tablespoon of sesame seeds on top of salad.

Serving suggestion: Toss with mixed greens, tomatoes, red onions, and additional diced oranges or kiwi.

*Fruit-flavored vinegars available at DrFuhrman.com.

PER SERVING: CALORIES 159; PROTEIN 4g; CARBOHYDRATES 16g; TOTAL FAT 9.6g; SATURATED FAT 1.5g; SODIUM 3mg; FIBER 3.5g; BETA-CAROTENE 62mcg; VITAMIN C 47mg; CALCIUM 128mg; IRON 2.2mg; FOLATE 38mcg; MAGNESIUM 74mg; ZINC 1.4mg; SELENIUM 3.2mcg

Pistachio Mint Dressing

Serves: 4

½ cup raw pistachio nuts
½ cup tightly packed fresh mint leaves
½ cup tightly packed fresh parsley leaves
2 cloves garlic, or to taste
2 scallions, coarsely chopped
½ cup soy, hemp, or almond milk, or as needed
1½ tablespoons champagne vinegar
1 tablespoon Dr. Fuhrman's Riesling Reserve Vinegar or other
   fruity vinegar
1 tablespoon nutritional yeast
Freshly ground black pepper, to taste

In a food processor, blend pistachios, mint, parsley, garlic, and
scallions to a fairly smooth paste. With the motor running, drizzle in
enough nondairy milk to achieve desired consistency. Add remaining
ingredients and process until well combined. Adjust seasonings, then
let stand for at least 1 hour so flavors mingle.

PER SERVING: CALORIES 127; PROTEIN 6g; CARBOHYDRATES 10g; TOTAL FAT 7.7g;
SATURATED FAT 0.9g; SODIUM 30mg; FIBER 3.7g; BETA-CAROTENE 303mcg; VITA-
MIN C 6mg; CALCIUM 74mg; IRON 3.6mg; FOLATE 95mcg; MAGNESIUM 39mg; ZINC
0.8mg; SELENIUM 4mcg

Russian Fig Dressing/Dip

Serves: 2

⅓ cup no-salt-added or low-sodium tomato sauce
⅓ cup raw almonds or 3 tablespoons raw almond butter
2 tablespoons raw sunflower seeds
3 tablespoons Dr. Fuhrman's Black Fig Vinegar or balsamic
  vinegar
1 tablespoon raisins or dried currants

Blend all ingredients in a food processor or high-powered blender until smooth.

PER SERVING: CALORIES 220; PROTEIN 5g; CARBOHYDRATES 19g; TOTAL FAT 14.2g; SATURATED FAT 1.3g; SODIUM 19mg; FIBER 4.2g; BETA-CAROTENE 151mcg; VITAMIN C 5mg; CALCIUM 69mg; IRON 1.8mg; FOLATE 31mcg; MAGNESIUM 88mg; ZINC 1.1mg; SELENIUM 6.3mcg

Southwest Ranch Dressing
Serves: 6

15 ounces silken tofu, drained and squeezed dry
⅓ cup white vinegar
2 tablespoons chia seeds
3 dates, pitted
¾ teaspoon ground coriander
½ teaspoon garlic powder
½ teaspoon onion powder
½ teaspoon black pepper
¼ teaspoon chipotle chili powder, or to taste
¼ cup minced tomatoes
2 tablespoons minced onion

Process all ingredients except tomatoes and onions in a high-powered blender until creamy. Adjust seasonings; you may want to add additional chili powder for a spicier dressing. Stir in minced tomatoes and onions.

PER SERVING: CALORIES 71; PROTEIN 4g; CARBOHYDRATES 7g; TOTAL FAT 3g; SATURATED FAT 0.5g; SODIUM 7mg; FIBER 1.9g; BETA-CAROTENE 50mcg; VITAMIN C 2mg; CALCIUM 74mg; IRON 0.8mg; FOLATE 7mcg; MAGNESIUM 35mg; ZINC 0.2mg; SELENIUM 0.3mcg

Walnut Vinaigrette Dressing

Serves: 4

¼ cup balsamic vinegar
½ cup water
¼ cup walnuts
¼ cup raisins
1 teaspoon Dijon mustard
1 clove garlic
¼ teaspoon dried thyme

Combine all ingredients in a high-powered blender.

PER SERVING: CALORIES 92; PROTEIN 1g; CARBOHYDRATES 11g; TOTAL FAT 4.8g; SATURATED FAT 0.5g; SODIUM 36mg; FIBER 0.9g; BETA-CAROTENE 3mcg; VITAMIN C 1mg; CALCIUM 20mg; IRON 0.6mg; FOLATE 8mcg; MAGNESIUM 17mg; ZINC 0.3mg; SELENIUM 0.5mcg

Super Simple Hummus

Serves: 4

1½ cups cooked garbanzo beans (chickpeas), or 1 (15-ounce) can
  no-salt-added or low-sodium garbanzo beans, drained
2 tablespoons lemon juice
2 tablespoons unhulled sesame seeds
1 clove garlic, minced
½ teaspoon ground cumin

Blend all ingredients in a high-powered blender or food processor.
Add 1–2 tablespoons water if desired, to adjust consistency. Can be
refrigerated in an airtight container for up to 5 days.

PER SERVING: CALORIES 131; PROTEIN 6g; CARBOHYDRATES 19g; TOTAL FAT 4g; SATURATED FAT 0.5g; SODIUM 6mg; FIBER 5.3g; BETA-CAROTENE 10mcg; VITAMIN C 5mg; CALCIUM 78mg; IRON 2.4mg; FOLATE 111mcg; MAGNESIUM 46mg; ZINC 1.3mg; SELENIUM 2.6mcg

Roasted Eggplant Hummus

Serves: 4

> 1 medium eggplant
> 1 bulb roasted garlic (see Note) or 8 cloves raw garlic
> 1 cup cooked garbanzo beans (chickpeas), or canned no-salt-
> added or low-sodium garbanzo beans, drained
> ⅓ cup water
> 4 tablespoons raw unhulled sesame seeds
> 2 tablespoons fresh lemon juice
> 1 tablespoon dried minced onions
> Dash paprika

Bake eggplant at 350°F for 45 minutes. Let cool; remove skin and discard. Blend all ingredients, including baked, peeled eggplant, in a food processor or high-powered blender until smooth and creamy. Serve with assorted raw vegetables.

Note: If using roasted garlic, roast garlic bulb along with eggplant for 15 minutes. Let cool, then squeeze garlic cloves out of bulb, removing the skin of the garlic.

PER SERVING: CALORIES 164; PROTEIN 7g; CARBOHYDRATES 24g; TOTAL FAT 5.8g; SATURATED FAT 0.8g; SODIUM 9mg; FIBER 9g; BETA-CAROTENE 29mcg; VITAMIN C 8mg; CALCIUM 132mg; IRON 2.9mg; FOLATE 113mcg; MAGNESIUM 74mg; ZINC 1.6mg; SELENIUM 2.9mcg

Fresh Tomato Salsa

Serves: 6

2 fresh tomatoes, chopped
1 small red onion, minced
2 scallions, minced
1 clove garlic, minced
½ jalapeño chili pepper, seeded and minced, or more to taste
3 tablespoons chopped cilantro
3 tablespoons fresh lime or lemon juice

In a mixing bowl, stir together all ingredients. Serve immediately or refrigerate in a tightly covered container for up to 5 days.

PER SERVING: CALORIES 15; PROTEIN 1g; CARBOHYDRATES 4g; TOTAL FAT 0.1g; SODIUM 4mg; FIBER 0.8g; BETA-CAROTENE 228mcg; VITAMIN C 8mg; CALCIUM 12mg; IRON 0.2mg; FOLATE 12mcg; MAGNESIUM 7mg; ZINC 0.1mg; SELENIUM 0.2mcg

Avocado Pumpkin Seed Salsa
Serves: 8

    1 red bell pepper
    1½ cups raw pumpkin seeds, toasted (see Note), divided
    2 tablespoons lime juice
    2 cloves garlic, minced
    1 jalapeño chili, minced
    3 large ripe avocados, cut into ½-inch dice
    ¼ cup cilantro leaves, chopped
    Freshly ground pepper

Broil pepper for 5 to 7 minutes, turning frequently until tender and skin is blackened. Transfer to a bowl with a tight-fitting lid or cover bowl with plastic wrap so pepper continues to soften and cool. When cooled and softened, peel off skin, stem and seed the pepper, then dice into ½-inch pieces.

Using a high-powered blender, grind ½ cup toasted pumpkin seeds into a coarse powder. In a medium bowl, mix the lime juice with the garlic, jalapeño, ground pumpkin seeds, diced bell pepper, avocados, cilantro, and remaining 1 cup toasted pumpkin seeds. Season with pepper and serve with romaine lettuce leaves, endive spears, or other raw vegetables.

Note: Toast pumpkin seeds in a large heavy skillet over medium high heat, stirring frequently, until seeds are puffed and beginning to brown, 2 to 4 minutes. Transfer to a large plate and cool.

PER SERVING: CALORIES 284; PROTEIN 9g; CARBOHYDRATES 15g; TOTAL FAT 23.4g; SATURATED FAT 4.5g; SODIUM 9mg; FIBER 7.9g; BETA-CAROTENE 453mcg; VITAMIN C 42mg; CALCIUM 27mg; IRON 4.2mg; FOLATE 64mcg; MAGNESIUM 169mg; ZINC 2.4mg; SELENIUM 1.6mcg

Mediterranean Tomato Spread

Serves: 4

> 1 cup cooked great northern beans, or canned no-salt-added
> or low-sodium great northern beans, drained
> 1 plum tomato
> ¼ cup pine nuts (see Note)
> 2 tablespoons unsulfured, unsalted dried tomatoes, minced
> 1 clove garlic
> 1 teaspoon Dr. Fuhrman's MatoZest* or other no-salt-added
> Italian seasoning blend
> 1 teaspoon Dr. Fuhrman's Black Fig Vinegar or balsamic vinegar
> ½ teaspoon minced rosemary, if desired

Combine all ingredients in a high-powered blender or food processor until smooth.

Note: Mediterranean stone pine nuts have better flavor and a higher protein content.

*A no-salt, dried tomato–based, garlicky Italian seasoning blend available at DrFuhrman.com.

PER SERVING: CALORIES 132; PROTEIN 7g; CARBOHYDRATES 15g; TOTAL FAT 6.1g; SATURATED FAT 0.5g; SODIUM 43mg; FIBER 3.6g; BETA-CAROTENE 179mcg; VITA-MIN C 3mg; CALCIUM 49mg; IRON 2.5mg; FOLATE 43mcg; MAGNESIUM 55mg; ZINC 1.2mg; SELENIUM 0.8mcg

Garlic Nutter Spread

Serves: 4

1 bulb garlic
1 cup raw cashews
6 tablespoons water
2 teaspoons nutritional yeast
⅛ teaspoon black pepper

Preheat oven to 350°F. Roast garlic in a small baking dish for about 25 minutes or until soft. When cool, cut top off garlic bulb and squeeze out soft cloves, discarding skins. Combine garlic and remaining ingredients in a high-powered blender. Blend until smooth.

This is a delicious and healthful condiment to have on hand to season cooked vegetable dishes or to add extra flavor to soups, sauces, and salad dressing ingredients.

PER SERVING: CALORIES 197; PROTEIN 7g; CARBOHYDRATES 11g; TOTAL FAT 15.1g; SATURATED FAT 2.7g; SODIUM 6mg; FIBER 1.6g; CALCIUM 16mg; IRON 2.7mg; FOLATE 55mcg; MAGNESIUM 103mg; ZINC 2.1mg; SELENIUM 7.4mcg

SALADS

Balsamic Tomato and Asparagus Salad
Serves: 4

1 pound asparagus, tough ends removed, cut into 2-inch pieces
1 cup cherry or grape tomatoes, cut in half
2 tablespoons balsamic vinegar
1 tablespoon orange juice
2 tablespoons minced red onion
Black pepper, to taste
5 ounces mixed baby greens
3 tablespoons pine nuts, half chopped and half left whole

Steam asparagus until just tender, about 12 minutes. Rinse with cold water to stop cooking; drain. Mix with tomatoes.

Combine vinegar, orange juice, red onion, and black pepper. Add to asparagus and tomatoes and toss to coat. Refrigerate for at least 15 minutes so flavors blend. Serve on a bed of baby greens. Sprinkle with pine nuts before serving.

PER SERVING: CALORIES 97; PROTEIN 6g; CARBOHYDRATES 10g; TOTAL FAT 4.7g; SATURATED FAT 0.4g; SODIUM 13mg; FIBER 3.9g; BETA-CAROTENE 749mcg; VITAMIN C 17mg; CALCIUM 55mg; IRON 3.2mg; FOLATE 103mcg; MAGNESIUM 45mg; ZINC 1.3mg; SELENIUM 2.7mcg

Kale Salad with Avocado and Apples

Serves: 4

> 1 bunch kale, tough stems and center ribs removed
> 1 avocado, peeled and chopped
> 2 tablespoons lemon juice
> 3 cloves garlic, minced
> 1 teaspoon fresh ginger root, minced
> ½ medium onion, minced
> 1 large apple, cored and chopped
> ½ cup raw cashews, chopped

Roll up each kale leaf and slice thinly. Add to bowl along with avocado and lemon juice. Using your hands, massage lemon juice and avocado into kale leaves until kale starts to soften and wilt and each leaf is coated, about 2 to 3 minutes. Mix in garlic, ginger, onion, and apple. Top with chopped cashews.

PER SERVING: CALORIES 319; PROTEIN 12g; CARBOHYDRATES 39g; TOTAL FAT 17.1g; SATURATED FAT 3.3g; SODIUM 92mg; FIBER 9.9g; BETA-CAROTENE 18,594mcg; VITA-MIN C 261mg; CALCIUM 297mg; IRON 4.7mg; FOLATE 101mcg; MAGNESIUM 135mg; ZINC 2.2mg; SELENIUM 4.2mcg

Kale and Quinoa Salad with Blueberries and Mangoes
Serves: 4

For the Salad:
    1 cup quinoa, rinsed well
    1½ cups shredded kale
    1 cup fresh blueberries
    1 cup cubed mango
    2 tablespoons chopped walnuts, toasted

For the Dressing:
    2 tablespoons balsamic vinegar
    2 tablespoons lemon juice
    ½ cup water
    ¼ cup walnuts
    ¼ cup raisins

Combine quinoa and 2 cups water in a medium saucepan. Bring to a boil. Cover, reduce heat to low, and simmer until water is absorbed and quinoa is translucent and tender, about 10 to 15 minutes. Fluff with a fork and transfer to a large bowl and let cool. Combine dressing ingredients in a high-powered blender. Mix quinoa with the dressing, kale, blueberries, mangoes, and walnuts.

PER SERVING: CALORIES 337; PROTEIN 13g; CARBOHYDRATES 57g; TOTAL FAT 10.1g; SATURATED FAT 1g; SODIUM 26mg; FIBER 5.7g; BETA-CAROTENE 2,515mcg; VITA-MIN C 46mg; CALCIUM 84mg; IRON 5.1mg; FOLATE 47mcg; MAGNESIUM 128mg; ZINC 1.9mg; SELENIUM 1.1mcg

Roasted Beets with Leafy Greens, Red Onions, and Walnuts

Serves: 2

2 medium red beets
¼ cup red wine vinegar
2 tablespoons raisins, finely chopped
1 tablespoon toasted caraway seeds, chopped
1 teaspoon garlic, finely chopped
10 cups Boston or green leaf lettuce
⅓ red onion, thinly sliced
¼ cup chopped walnuts

Roast beets at 350°F for 50 minutes or until tender when pierced. Let cool and peel off skins. Slice beets thinly and marinate in red wine vinegar, chopped raisins, toasted caraway seeds, and chopped garlic for at least 1 hour. In a large salad bowl, toss beet and vinegar mixture with remaining ingredients.

PER SERVING: CALORIES 219; PROTEIN 8g; CARBOHYDRATES 27g; TOTAL FAT 10.8g; SATURATED FAT 1g; SODIUM 83mg; FIBER 8.2g; BETA-CAROTENE 5,489mcg; VITA-MIN C 17mg; CALCIUM 159mg; IRON 5.4mg; FOLATE 309mcg; MAGNESIUM 92mg; ZINC 1.5mg; SELENIUM 3.7mcg

Warm Corn and Zucchini Salad with Mint
Serves: 4

⅓ cup low-sodium or no-salt-added vegetable broth, or more if
   needed to achieve desired consistency
1 cup diced onion
2 teaspoons or 4 cloves minced garlic
2 cups diced zucchini
2 cups fresh corn kernels
¼ teaspoon ground cumin
¼ teaspoon ground coriander
3 tablespoons chopped fresh mint
1 tablespoon fresh lemon juice
Freshly ground black pepper, to taste

Heat vegetable broth in a large sauté pan. Add onion, garlic, zucchini,
and corn and sauté for 10 minutes or until vegetables are tender. Add
cumin and coriander and continue cooking until liquid is evaporated.
Remove from heat. Add mint, lemon juice, and pepper.

PER SERVING: CALORIES 333; PROTEIN 9g; CARBOHYDRATES 68g; TOTAL FAT 4.1g;
SATURATED FAT 0.6g; SODIUM 38mg; FIBER 1.5g; BETA-CAROTENE 69mcg; VITAMIN C
15mg; CALCIUM 31mg; IRON 2.6mg; FOLATE 26mcg; MAGNESIUM 121mg; ZINC
2.1mg; SELENIUM 13.4mcg

SOUPS

Black Bean Quinoa Soup

Serves: 4

> 1 medium onion, chopped
> 1 green bell pepper, chopped
> 4 cloves garlic, minced
> 1 cup chopped fresh tomato
> 1 teaspoon ground cumin
> 2 teaspoons chili powder
> ¼ teaspoon crushed red pepper flakes
> 1 large carrot, chopped
> 5 cups low-sodium or no-salt-added vegetable broth
> ½ cup quinoa, rinsed
> 3 cups cooked black beans, or 2 (15-ounce) cans low-sodium or
>   no-salt-added black beans, drained
> 4 cups baby spinach
> ¼ cup chopped cilantro
> 1 tablespoon fresh lime juice
> 1 avocado, chopped

In a soup pot, heat 2–3 tablespoons water, add onion and green pepper and water-sauté about 5 minutes, until tender, adding more water if needed to prevent sticking. Add garlic and sauté another 30 seconds, until fragrant. Add the fresh tomato, cumin, chili powder, and red pepper flakes and cook for 2–3 minutes, until tomatoes soften. Add carrots and vegetable broth, bring to a boil, stir in the quinoa, reduce heat, and cover and cook for 10 minutes. Add black beans and continue cooking until heated through and quinoa is tender, about 10 minutes. Add spinach and stir until wilted. Remove from heat and stir in cilantro and lime juice. Serve garnished with chopped avocado.

PER SERVING: CALORIES 419; PROTEIN 25g; CARBOHYDRATES 63g; TOTAL FAT 10.9g; SATURATED FAT 1.8g; SODIUM 151mg; FIBER 18.7g; BETA-CAROTENE 3,671mcg; VITAMIN C 51mg; CALCIUM 133mg; IRON 7mg; FOLATE 323mcg; MAGNESIUM 191mg; ZINC 3.1mg; SELENIUM 2.7mcg

Boston Green Pea Soup

Serves: 2

1 medium onion, diced
3 cups no-salt-added or low-sodium vegetable broth
10 ounces frozen peas
1 head Boston lettuce, coarsely chopped
⅛ teaspoon black pepper
⅛ teaspoon dried tarragon leaves
½ cup unsweetened soy, almond, or hemp milk
1 tablespoon fresh lemon juice

Heat 2–3 tablespoons water in a soup pot. Add onions and water-sauté until tender, about 5 minutes. Stir in vegetable broth, peas, lettuce, pepper, and tarragon; bring to a boil, reduce heat, and simmer for 10 minutes. Stir in nondairy milk. Blend soup in a blender until smooth, working in batches. Pour blended soup into a large bowl after each batch, and when all the soup is blended, return to soup pot and heat through. Stir in lemon juice and remove from heat.

PER SERVING: CALORIES 224; PROTEIN 18g; CARBOHYDRATES 33g; TOTAL FAT 3.7g; SATURATED FAT 0.9g; SODIUM 247mg; FIBER 9.6g; BETA-CAROTENE 2,215mcg; VITAMIN C 22mg; CALCIUM 86mg; IRON 3.7mg; FOLATE 107mcg; MAGNESIUM 56mg; ZINC 1.7mg; SELENIUM 4.6mcg

Creamy Cabbage Soup

Serves: 4

1 head cabbage, cut into pieces
3 medium carrots, coarsely chopped
1 cup celery, coarsely chopped
2 leeks, coarsely chopped
2 cloves garlic, minced
1 tablespoon Dr. Fuhrman's VegiZest or other no-salt seasoning blend, adjusted to taste
2 cups carrot juice
6 cups low-sodium or no-salt-added vegetable broth
½ teaspoon nutmeg
⅛ teaspoon cayenne pepper, or to taste
5 cups chopped kale leaves or baby spinach
1 cup raw cashews, or ½ cup raw cashew butter

Place all the ingredients except the cashews in a pot. Cover and simmer for 30 minutes or until vegetables are tender. In a food processor or high-powered blender, blend two-thirds of the soup liquid and vegetables with the cashews until smooth and creamy. Return to the pot.

PER SERVING: CALORIES 393; PROTEIN 18g; CARBOHYDRATES 56g; TOTAL FAT 16.4g; SATURATED FAT 3g; SODIUM 192mg; FIBER 11.9g; BETA-CAROTENE 23,401mcg; VITAMIN C 203mg; CALCIUM 305mg; IRON 6.6mg; FOLATE 180mcg; MAGNESIUM 196mg; ZINC 3.2mg; SELENIUM 9.8mcg

Creamy Butternut Ginger Soup

Serves: 5

2 cups water
2 cups unsweetened soy, hemp, or almond milk
3 cups no-salt-added or low-sodium vegetable broth
3 carrots, sliced in 1–2-inch slices
5 celery stalks, sliced in 1–2-inch slices
2 onions, cut in half
2 teaspoons minced peeled ginger
2 butternut squash, peeled and cubed
10 ounces shiitake, cremini, or oyster mushrooms, stems
   trimmed, and sliced
1½ cups cooked great northern beans, or 1 (15-ounce) can
   no-salt-added or low-sodium great northern beans, drained
⅛ teaspoon cayenne pepper, or to taste
6 ounces baby kale or baby spinach

Place water, nondairy milk, vegetable broth, carrots, celery, onions, ginger, and butternut squash in a large soup pot. Bring to a boil, reduce heat, and simmer for 30 minutes or until squash is tender. Place soup in a food processor or blender, and, working in batches, blend until smooth. Return to pot. Add mushrooms, beans, and cayenne pepper; bring to a simmer and cook for 20 minutes. Add baby kale or spinach and continue cooking until greens are wilted.

PER SERVING: CALORIES 318; PROTEIN 19g; CARBOHYDRATES 60g; TOTAL FAT 3.8g; SATURATED FAT 0.7g; SODIUM 188mg; FIBER 12.8g; BETA-CAROTENE 16,098mcg; VITAMIN C 96mg; CALCIUM 287mg; IRON 6.1mg; FOLATE 168mcg; MAGNESIUM 167mg; ZINC 2.3mg; SELENIUM 12.4mcg

Greens, Beans, and Mushroom Stew

Serves: 6

1½ cups chopped onions
3 cloves garlic, chopped
1 cup chopped carrots
1 cup chopped celery
5 cups assorted mushrooms (button, portobello, and/or shiitake), chopped
2 cups lentils
3 cups low-sodium or no-salt-added vegetable broth
3 cups chopped tomatoes
¼ cup tomato paste
1 tablespoon cider vinegar
2 teaspoons paprika
1½ teaspoons cumin
2 teaspoons fennel seed
½ teaspoon ground black pepper
¼ teaspoon cayenne pepper
1 cup chopped green bell pepper
10 ounces turnip greens or mustard greens, tough stems removed, chopped

Heat 2 tablespoons water and water-sauté onions, garlic, carrots, and celery until starting to soften. Add mushrooms and continue cooking until mushrooms lose their water. Add lentils, vegetable broth, chopped tomatoes, tomato paste, vinegar, paprika, cumin, fennel seed, black pepper, and cayenne pepper. Simmer covered until lentils are tender and most of the liquid is absorbed, 25 to 30 minutes. Add green pepper during the last 10 minutes of cooking. Add greens and cook until wilted.

If stew appears too dry, add additional water or vegetable broth.

PER SERVING: CALORIES 323; PROTEIN 25g; CARBOHYDRATES 58g; TOTAL FAT 1.8g; SATURATED FAT 0.2g; SODIUM 71mg; FIBER 26.2g; BETA-CAROTENE 5,486mcg; VITAMIN C 77mg; CALCIUM 146mg; IRON 7.1mg; FOLATE 443mcg; MAGNESIUM 132mg; ZINC 4mg; SELENIUM 14.3mcg

In-a-Hurry Anticancer Soup
Serves: 6

   3 large onions, chopped
   5 large zucchini, cut into 1-inch pieces
   2 cups mushrooms, any type, chopped
   1 pound kale, tough stems removed, chopped
   1 pound mustard greens, tough stems removed, chopped
   1 (15-ounce) can low-sodium or no-salt-added adzuki beans
   6 cups carrot juice*
   2 cups water
   1 tablespoon Dr. Fuhrman's VegiZest or other no-salt seasoning
     blend, adjusted to taste
   ½ cup raw cashews

Place all ingredients except cashews in a large stock pot. Bring to a boil, then reduce heat to a simmer; cover and cook for 30 minutes or until the vegetables are soft. Add cooked soup and cashews to a food processor or high-powered blender and blend until smooth and creamy. For a chunky soup, blend only a portion of the cooked soup and then return to pot.

*For speed in preparation, this recipe uses a store-bought refrigerated carrot juice.

PER SERVING: CALORIES 335; PROTEIN 17g; CARBOHYDRATES 60g; TOTAL FAT 6.6g; SATURATED FAT 1.2g; SODIUM 153mg; FIBER 12.1g; BETA-CAROTENE 34,089mcg; VITAMIN C 197mg; CALCIUM 322mg; IRON 6.9mg; FOLATE 275mcg; MAGNESIUM 181mg; ZINC 2.9mg; SELENIUM 9.2mcg

White Bean and Kale Soup

Serves: 4

    8 cups low-sodium or no-salt-added vegetable broth, divided
    8 large cloves garlic, minced
    1 medium onion, chopped
    8 cups chopped kale
    4½ cups cooked white beans, or 3 (15-ounce) cans no-salt-added
        or low-sodium white beans, drained, divided
    4 plum tomatoes, chopped
    1 teaspoon dried oregano
    ½ teaspoon dried basil
    ½ teaspoon dried thyme
    ½ cup chopped parsley
    Black pepper, to taste

In a large pot, heat 2–3 tablespoons of vegetable broth and sauté
garlic and onion until soft. Add kale, 6 cups of the vegetable broth,
2 cups of the beans, tomatoes, herbs, and pepper. Simmer for 5
minutes. In a blender or food processor, blend the remaining broth
and beans until smooth. Stir into the soup. Simmer for 30 minutes or
until kale is very tender.

PER SERVING: CALORIES 367; PROTEIN 29g; CARBOHYDRATES 62g; TOTAL FAT 3.8g;
SATURATED FAT 1.0g; SODIUM 178mg; FIBER 13.7g; BETA-CAROTENE 10,433mcg;
VITAMIN C 146mg; CALCIUM 340mg; IRON 9.5mg; FOLATE 184mcg; MAGNESIUM
155mg; ZINC 3mg; SELENIUM 3.9mcg

MAIN DISHES AND VEGETABLE SIDE DISHES

Baja Mango Black Bean Lettuce Wraps
Serves: 4

> 2 cups cooked black beans, or canned no-salt-added or low-sodium black beans, drained
> ½ large ripe avocado, peeled, pitted, and mashed
> 4 cloves roasted garlic, mashed
> ⅓ cup fresh tomatoes, chopped
> ½ medium green bell pepper, seeded and chopped
> 1 mango, diced
> 2 red radishes, diced
> 1 jalapeño pepper, diced and seeded
> 3 green onions, chopped
> ⅓ cup chopped fresh cilantro
> 2 tablespoons fresh lime juice
> 1 teaspoon ground cumin
> 8 large romaine or Boston lettuce leaves

In a bowl, mash together beans, avocado, and garlic with a fork until well blended and only slightly chunky. Add all ingredients except the lettuce, and mix. Place approximately ¼ cup of the mixture in the center of each lettuce leaf and roll up like a burrito.

PER SERVING: CALORIES 221; PROTEIN 11g; CARBOHYDRATES 39g; TOTAL FAT 4.5g; SATURATED FAT 0.7g; SODIUM 21mg; FIBER 13.4g; BETA-CAROTENE 4,520mcg; VITAMIN C 66mg; CALCIUM 92mg; IRON 3.5mg; FOLATE 321mcg; MAGNESIUM 95mg; ZINC 1.5mg; SELENIUM 2.4mcg

Balsamic Portobello and Eggplant Stacks

Serves: 4

    4 portobello mushrooms
    ¼ cup balsamic vinegar
    1 medium eggplant, sliced ⅓ inch thick
    ¼ cup fresh basil leaves
    1 tomato, sliced ⅓ inch thick
    ½ teaspoon oregano
    ¼ teaspoon black pepper
    1½ cups no-salt-added or low-sodium pasta sauce
    ¼ cup pine nuts, toasted and chopped (see Note)

Preheat oven to 350°F. Marinate mushrooms in balsamic vinegar for 10 minutes. Remove from marinade. On a nonstick baking pan, layer in 4 stacks: mushrooms, eggplant, basil leaves, and tomato. Season with oregano and black pepper. Bake for 30 minutes or until mushrooms and eggplant are soft. In a small saucepan, heat pasta sauce. Serve stacks topped with sauce and chopped pine nuts.

Note: Mediterranean stone pine nuts have better flavor and a higher protein content.

PER SERVING: CALORIES 218; PROTEIN 6g; CARBOHYDRATES 29g; TOTAL FAT 10.8g; SATURATED FAT 1.1g; SODIUM 37mg; FIBER 8.6g; BETA-CAROTENE 586mcg; VITA-MIN C 18mg; CALCIUM 55mg; IRON 1.9mg; FOLATE 55mcg; MAGNESIUM 73mg; ZINC 1.2mg; SELENIUM 3.2mcg

Bean Pasta with Cauliflower in a Garlicky Walnut Sauce

Serves: 6

7 ounces bean pasta (see Note), cooked according to package
directions and set aside
1 pound fresh or frozen cauliflower florets, steamed
Squeeze of lemon

For the Sauce:

7 cloves garlic, peeled, divided
2 cups unsweetened almond or soy milk
1 cup walnuts, toasted
1 no-salt-added vegan bouillon cube, or 2 tablespoons
    Dr. Fuhrman's VegiZest
¼ teaspoon ground nutmeg
3 tablespoons nutritional yeast
1 pound fresh or frozen spinach, chopped
1 tablespoon dried marjoram, or 1½ tablespoons chopped fresh
    marjoram (or substitute dried or fresh oregano)

To prepare sauce, roast 6 cloves of the garlic in oven-proof dish, with
almond milk to cover, for 30 minutes at 350°F, covering the dish with
foil. In a high-powered blender, puree walnuts, bouillon or VegiZest,
nutmeg, and yeast with remaining almond milk and roasted garlic
and remaining clove of raw garlic until smooth; transfer to a medium
saucepan. Bring to a boil and simmer for 5 minutes until sauce thickens
slightly. Stir in chopped spinach and marjoram and keep warm.

Divide the pasta among 6 plates, ladle on the sauce, and top with
cauliflower florets and a squeeze of lemon. Serve immediately.

This may also be made with pistachios instead of walnuts for a
delicious twist on the classic Italian walnut sauce.

Non-vegan option: Add 4 ounces shredded cooked chicken to the sauce.

Note: Explore Asian brand makes several varieties of bean pasta.

PER SERVING: CALORIES 290; PROTEIN 17g; CARBOHYDRATES 28g; TOTAL FAT 15.1g;
SATURATED FAT 1.6g; SODIUM 153mg; FIBER 9.5g; BETA-CAROTENE 5,170mcg; VITA-
MIN C 61mg; CALCIUM 192mg; IRON 6.8mg; FOLATE 390mcg; MAGNESIUM 151mg;
ZINC 2.5mg; SELENIUM 8.8mcg

California Creamed Kale

Serves: 4

  2 bunches kale, leaves removed from tough stems
  1 cup raw cashews
  1 cup unsweetened soy, hemp, or almond milk
  4 tablespoons onion flakes
  1 tablespoon Dr. Fuhrman's VegiZest or other no-salt seasoning
    blend, adjusted to taste

Place kale in a large steamer pot and steam 13 minutes until soft. Meanwhile, place remaining ingredients in a high-powered blender and blend until smooth. Place kale in a colander and press to remove some of the excess water. In a bowl, coarsely chop and mix kale with the cream sauce.

Note: This sauce may be used with broccoli, spinach, or other steamed vegetables.

PER SERVING: CALORIES 279; PROTEIN 12g; CARBOHYDRATES 26g; TOTAL FAT 16.7g; SATURATED FAT 2.9g; SODIUM 79mg; FIBER 3.8g; BETA-CAROTENE 7,060mcg; VITA-MIN C 90mg; CALCIUM 144mg; IRON 4.4mg; FOLATE 47mcg; MAGNESIUM 144mg; ZINC 2.7mg; SELENIUM 10.6mcg

Chickpea and Tofu Curry

Serves: 3

> 3 prunes, chopped and soaked in 2 tablespoons water for
>   30 minutes
> 1 medium onion, chopped
> 1 clove garlic, minced
> 1 teaspoon ground cumin
> 1 teaspoon curry powder
> ½ teaspoon ground black pepper
> 8 ounces firm tofu, cut into cubes
> 1½ cups cooked chickpeas, or 1 (15-ounce) can no-salt-added
>   or low-sodium chickpeas, drained
> ½ cup water
> 2 tomatoes, chopped
> 6 ounces fresh spinach

Remove prunes from soaking water and chop more. Add prunes and the soaking water to a large skillet, bring water to a simmer, and then add onion and garlic. Sauté onion and garlic until tender. Stir in cumin, curry powder, and black pepper. Add cubed tofu and cook for 1 minute, stirring constantly. Add chickpeas and water and simmer for 5 minutes. Add tomatoes and spinach and continue to cook until spinach is wilted, about 3 minutes.

PER SERVING: CALORIES 315; PROTEIN 24g; CARBOHYDRATES 41g; TOTAL FAT 9.4g; SATURATED FAT 1.3g; SODIUM 70mg; FIBER 12g; BETA-CAROTENE 3,609mcg; VITAMIN C 31mg; CALCIUM 647mg; IRON 6.6mg; FOLATE 294mcg; MAGNESIUM 147mg; ZINC 3mg; SELENIUM 17.2mcg

Black-Eyed Collards

Serves: 6

> 1 cup low-sodium or no-salt-added vegetable broth
> 1 large onion, sliced
> ½ pound collard greens, washed and chopped
> ¼ cup currants or raisins
> 1½ cups cooked black-eyed peas,* or 1 (15-ounce) can
>   low-sodium or no-salt-added black-eyed peas, drained
> ⅛ teaspoon hot pepper flakes, or more to taste

Heat 2–3 tablespoons of the vegetable broth in a large skillet; add onion slices and sauté until tender. Add collards, remaining vegetable broth, and currants or raisins; bring to a boil, reduce heat, cover, and cook for 5 minutes or until collards are tender. Stir in black-eyed peas and hot pepper flakes and heat through.

*You can substitute any white bean for black-eyed peas.

PER SERVING: CALORIES 99; PROTEIN 6g; CARBOHYDRATES 20g; TOTAL FAT 0.4g; SATURATED FAT 0.1g; SODIUM 13mg; FIBER 4.7g; BETA-CAROTENE 1,461mcg; VITA-MIN C 15mg; CALCIUM 104mg; IRON 1.9mg; FOLATE 103mcg; MAGNESIUM 36mg; ZINC 0.7mg; SELENIUM 1.2mcg

Stuffed Eggplant Tofenade

Serves: 4

  1 cup shelled edamame, fresh or frozen
  ¼ cup extra firm tofu
  ⅓ cup water
  4 tablespoons raw pumpkin seeds, toasted
  ½ teaspoon dried basil
  ½ teaspoon dried oregano
  ⅛ teaspoon black pepper
  1 medium red bell pepper, coarsely chopped
  1 medium onion, coarsely chopped
  ½ cup coarsely chopped carrots
  4 cloves garlic, chopped
  4 ounces baby spinach
  2 medium eggplants, peeled and sliced lengthwise into
    ¼-inch slices
  2 cups no-salt-added or low-sodium pasta sauce

Preheat oven to 350°F. Boil edamame for 5 minutes. Combine in food processor with tofu, water, pumpkin seeds, basil, oregano, and black pepper. Set aside.

In 2 tablespoons water, sauté red peppers, onion, carrots, and garlic until tender, adding more water if needed. Add spinach and cook until wilted. Set aside.

Roast eggplant in baking pan lightly oiled with olive oil for about 20 minutes, or until tender and flexible enough to roll up. In baking pan, spread about ¼ cup tomato sauce. Place 1–2 tablespoons edamame puree in center of each eggplant slice. Top with sautéed vegetable mixture. Roll up and place in baking dish, seam side down. Top with remaining sauce. Bake 20 to 30 minutes or until heated through.

PER SERVING: CALORIES 356; PROTEIN 16g; CARBOHYDRATES 50g; TOTAL FAT 14.2g; SATURATED FAT 2.2g; SODIUM 85mg; FIBER 18.2g; BETA-CAROTENE 3,868mcg; VITA-MIN C 73mg; CALCIUM 250mg; IRON 5.3mg; FOLATE 285mcg; MAGNESIUM 181mg; ZINC 2.5mg; SELENIUM 6.3mcg

Mexican Lentils

Serves: 4

1 cup lentils, uncooked
1 cup frozen or fresh corn
1 cup tomato sauce, no salt added
1 medium onion, chopped
½ teaspoon cumin powder
1 teaspoon chili powder
2 tablespoons fresh cilantro

Boil lentils in 2 cups water for 30 minutes and then drain. Add corn, tomato sauce, onion, cumin powder, and chili powder; simmer over low heat for 20 minutes. Stir in cilantro.

Serving suggestion: Serve stuffed into poblano chili peppers. Cut 3–4 peppers in half lengthwise, fill with lentil mixture, and bake at 350°F for 30 minutes.

PER SERVING: CALORIES 241; PROTEIN 15g; CARBOHYDRATES 45g; TOTAL FAT 1.0g; SATURATED FAT 0.1g; SODIUM 14mg; FIBER 17.1g; BETA-CAROTENE 243mcg; VITA-MIN C 16mg; CALCIUM 47mg; IRON 4.4mg; FOLATE 257mcg; MAGNESIUM 81mg; ZINC 2.6mg; SELENIUM 4.8mcg

Portobellos and Beans

Serves: 2

1 large onion, chopped
2 garlic cloves, chopped
2 large portobello mushroom caps, sliced thin
½ cup red wine or low-sodium vegetable broth
1 large tomato, diced, or 8 halved cherry tomatoes
1½ cups cooked garbanzo beans, or 1 (15-ounce) can no-salt-
added or low-sodium garbanzo beans, drained

Water-sauté onion and garlic for 2 minutes, or until onions are soft. Add mushrooms and red wine or broth and continue cooking for 5 minutes until mushrooms are tender. Add tomatoes and garbanzo beans. Simmer for 5 minutes.

PER SERVING: CALORIES 326; PROTEIN 20g; CARBOHYDRATES 51g; TOTAL FAT 3.9g; SATURATED FAT 0.4g; SODIUM 26mg; FIBER 13.2g; BETA-CAROTENE 828mcg; VITAMIN C 31mg; CALCIUM 103mg; IRON 4.8mg; FOLATE 261mcg; MAGNESIUM 99mg; ZINC 2.8mg; SELENIUM 12.1mcg

Ratatouille over Spaghetti Squash

Serves: 4

1 medium spaghetti squash
1 medium onion, chopped
2 cloves garlic, chopped
2 large tomatoes, chopped
1 medium eggplant, peeled and cubed
1 medium zucchini, chopped
1 red pepper, chopped
1 cup sliced mushrooms
1 teaspoon oregano
1 teaspoon basil
1½ cups no-salt-added or low-sodium spaghetti sauce

Preheat oven to 350°F. Slice spaghetti squash in half lengthwise and remove seeds. Place both halves, skin side up, on a baking sheet. Bake for 45 minutes or until tender.

Meanwhile, heat 2 tablespoons water in a large deep skillet. Water-sauté onion until softened, about 3 minutes. Add garlic and cook for 1 minute, adding more water as necessary to prevent scorching. Reduce heat to low-medium and add tomatoes, eggplant, zucchini, red pepper, mushrooms, oregano, and basil. Cover and cook, stirring occasionally until vegetables are very tender, about 1 hour. Add spaghetti sauce and simmer for an additional 5 minutes.

When squash is done, remove from oven and, using a fork, scrape spaghetti-like strands from the squash onto serving plates. Top with eggplant mixture.

PER SERVING: CALORIES 288; PROTEIN 9g; CARBOHYDRATES 56g; TOTAL FAT 7.2g; SATURATED FAT 1.1g; SODIUM 101mg; FIBER 10.4g; BETA-CAROTENE 1,209mcg; VITAMIN C 78mg; CALCIUM 155mg; IRON 3mg; FOLATE 131mcg; MAGNESIUM 109mg; ZINC 1.6mg; SELENIUM 5.2mcg

Sweet and Smoky Baked Beans

Serves: 4

1 large onion, chopped
4 cloves garlic, chopped
1 cup low-sodium or no-salt-added tomato sauce
1 apple, cored and quartered
¼ cup raisins, soaked in hot water to cover for 30 minutes
1 tablespoon apple cider vinegar
2 tablespoons prepared mustard, no salt added or low sodium
1 teaspoon Bragg Liquid Aminos
1 teaspoon chipotle chili powder
3 cups cooked red kidney beans, or 2 (15-ounce) cans low-sodium or no-salt-added red kidney beans, drained

Preheat oven to 350°F. Water-sauté onions and garlic in 2–3 tablespoons water until tender, about 5 minutes. Add small amounts of additional water as needed to prevent burning.

Blend tomato sauce, apple, raisins and soaking water, vinegar, mustard, Bragg Liquid Aminos, and chipotle chili powder in a high-powered blender until smooth. Combine kidney beans, blended mixture, and sautéed onions in a large casserole dish. Cover and bake for 50 minutes.

PER SERVING: CALORIES 249; PROTEIN 15g; CARBOHYDRATES 49g; TOTAL FAT 0.6g; SATURATED FAT 0.1g; SODIUM 121mg; FIBER 15.1g; BETA-CAROTENE 138mcg; VITAMIN C 14mg; CALCIUM 88mg; IRON 5mg; FOLATE 111mcg; MAGNESIUM 77mg; ZINC 1.5mg; SELENIUM 4mcg

Sweet Potatoes Topped with Black Beans and Kale

Serves: 4

   4 medium sweet potatoes
   1 onion, chopped
   2 cloves garlic, chopped
   6 cups chopped kale
   1½ cups cooked black beans, or 1 (15-ounce) can no-salt-added
      or low-sodium black beans, drained
   1½ cups diced tomatoes
   2 teaspoons chili powder
   1 teaspoon cumin
   2 tablespoons chopped cilantro
   1 cup unsweetened nondairy yogurt

Pierce sweet potatoes in several spots with a fork. Microwave on high until soft, 12–16 minutes. Potatoes can also be baked in a 350°F oven for 50 minutes or until soft.

Meanwhile, heat 2 tablespoons water in a large pan and water-sauté onion and garlic for 2 minutes. Add kale and stir until wilted. Cover pan and cook until kale is tender, adding water as needed, about 10 minutes. Add black beans, tomatoes, chili powder, and cumin; bring to a simmer and cook for 5 minutes.

Cut each potato lengthwise, skin and partially mash, then top with bean mixture. Sprinkle with cilantro. Top with nondairy yogurt.

PER SERVING: CALORIES 342; PROTEIN 16g; CARBOHYDRATES 69g; TOTAL FAT 2.8g; SATURATED FAT 0.4g; SODIUM 159mg; FIBER 13.7g; BETA-CAROTENE 20,928mcg; VITAMIN C 138mg; CALCIUM 295mg; IRON 5mg; FOLATE 162mcg; MAGNESIUM 151mg; ZINC 2mg; SELENIUM 11.4mcg

Szechuan Sesame Stir-Fry

Serves: 4

For the Sauce:
- ¼ cup unhulled sesame seeds, lightly pan toasted
- 1 cup unsweetened soy, hemp, or almond milk
- 6 Medjool or 12 Deglet Noor dates, pitted
- ½ tablespoon minced ginger
- 4 cloves garlic, peeled
- ¼ teaspoon red pepper flakes, or to taste

For the Stir-Fry:
- 2 cups broccoli florets
- 1½ cups cauliflower florets
- 1 red bell pepper, cut into 1-inch pieces
- 1½ cups sliced shiitake mushrooms
- 1 cup fresh snow peas
- ½ cup baby corn, each broken in half
- 2 cups cooked brown, black, or wild rice

In a high-powered blender, puree all sauce ingredients until smooth. Set aside.

Heat ¼ cup water in a wok or large sauté pan. Add broccoli and cauliflower; cover and steam for 8 minutes. Remove cover and add bell pepper, mushrooms, snow peas, and corn and stir-fry for an additional 5 minutes or until vegetables are crisp-tender. Add small amounts of water as needed to prevent sticking. Add sauce to veggies and continue to stir-fry for 1–2 minutes to heat through. Serve over rice.

Non-vegan option: Top with 8 ounces broiled scallops or pieces of broiled wild salmon.

PER SERVING: CALORIES 411; PROTEIN 14g; CARBOHYDRATES 82g; TOTAL FAT 6.8g; SATURATED FAT 0.9g; SODIUM 75mg; FIBER 10.3g; BETA-CAROTENE 1,004mcg; VITAMIN C 107mg; CALCIUM 175mg; IRON 4.5mg; FOLATE 126mcg; MAGNESIUM 147mg; ZINC 3.7mg; SELENIUM 22.6mcg

Tailgate Chili with Black and Red Beans

Serves: 5

½ cup bulgur

1 cup water

3 cups chopped onions

3 cloves garlic, minced or pressed

2 green bell peppers, chopped

3 cups diced tomatoes

1½ cups cooked black beans, or 1 (15-ounce) can no-salt-added
    or low-sodium black beans, drained

3 cups cooked red kidney beans, or 2 (15-ounce) cans no-salt-
    added or low-sodium red kidney beans, drained

2 cups fresh or frozen corn kernels

2 tablespoons chili powder

2 teaspoons ground cumin

¼ cup chopped fresh cilantro

Combine bulgur and water in a saucepan. Bring to a boil, reduce heat, and simmer for 12 to 15 minutes or until tender.

While bulgur cooks, heat 2 tablespoons water in a large saucepan and water-sauté onions and garlic until almost soft, about 5 minutes. Stir in green peppers and sauté an additional 3 minutes, adding more water as needed. Stir in diced tomatoes, beans, corn, chili powder, and cumin. Bring to a boil, reduce heat, cover, and simmer for 20 minutes. Add bulgur and simmer for an additional 5 minutes. Stir in cilantro.

PER SERVING: CALORIES 394; PROTEIN 23g; CARBOHYDRATES 79g; TOTAL FAT 2.6g; SATURATED FAT 0.5g; SODIUM 54mg; FIBER 20.7g; BETA-CAROTENE 1,221mcg; VITA-MIN C 68mg; CALCIUM 120mg; IRON 5.3mg; FOLATE 287mcg; MAGNESIUM 149mg; ZINC 2.7mg; SELENIUM 3.5mcg

Vegetable Gumbo
Serves: 4

   1 medium green pepper, chopped
   1 medium red pepper, chopped
   ½ large onion, thinly sliced
   1 cup chopped celery
   2 cloves garlic, minced
   1 cup plus 2–3 tablespoons no-salt-added or low-sodium
      vegetable broth
   10 ounces fresh mushrooms, sliced
   1 zucchini, chopped
   1 cup frozen okra, defrosted and sliced
   1½ cups diced tomatoes
   1½ cups cooked kidney beans, or 1 (15-ounce) can low-sodium
      or no-salt-added kidney beans, drained
   2 cups chopped collard greens
   1 tablespoon lemon juice
   1 teaspoon dried oregano
   1 teaspoon dried basil
   ¼ teaspoon red pepper flakes, or to taste
   2 cups cooked brown rice, wild rice, or quinoa

Sauté green and red pepper, onion, celery, and garlic in 2–3 tablespoons vegetable broth until tender. Add mushrooms and zucchini and cook until liquid is evaporated. Stir in okra, tomatoes, beans, collard greens, remaining vegetable broth, lemon juice, oregano, basil, and red pepper flakes. (Add more red pepper flakes if you like it spicy.) Bring to a boil, reduce heat, and then cover and simmer for 10 minutes or until vegetables are tender. Serve on top of rice or quinoa.

Non-vegan option: Add 4 ounces of cooked shredded chicken or small wild-caught, domestic shrimp during the last few minutes of cooking time.

PER SERVING: CALORIES 266; PROTEIN 15g; CARBOHYDRATES 53g; TOTAL FAT 1.9g; SATURATED FAT 0.3g; SODIUM 39mg; FIBER 10.8g; BETA-CAROTENE 565mcg; VITAMIN C 63mg; CALCIUM 123mg; IRON 3.4mg; FOLATE 223mcg; MAGNESIUM 127mg; ZINC 2.3mg; SELENIUM 46.2mcg

Vegetable Chickpea Loaf
Serves: 8

½ cup walnuts

1½ cups cooked chickpeas, or 1 (15-ounce) can no-salt-added or
    low-sodium chickpeas, drained

1 medium onion, quartered

1 medium carrot, cut into 1-inch pieces

1 medium green bell pepper, seeded and cut into large chunks

1 cup sliced mushrooms

1 cup cooked brown rice

2 tablespoons arrowroot powder

2 teaspoons agar powder (see Box)

1½ tablespoons stone-ground mustard

1 tablespoon nutritional yeast

¼ teaspoon dried thyme

⅛ teaspoon dried sage

⅛ teaspoon dried marjoram

⅛ teaspoon black pepper

½ cup low-sodium ketchup, for top of loaf

Preheat oven to 350°F. Place walnuts and chickpeas in a food processor
and process until finely chopped. Transfer to a large mixing bowl.

Add onion, carrot, bell pepper, and mushrooms to the food processor
and process until finely chopped. Add to the chickpea mixture. Add
to this mixture rice, arrowroot powder, agar powder, mustard, nutritional yeast, thyme, sage, marjoram, and black pepper and mix well.

Lightly wipe a 5-by-9-inch loaf pan with olive oil. Place mixture
into pan, patting into place. Top with ketchup. Bake for 50 minutes.
Let stand for 30 minutes before slicing; loaf will firm up as it cools.
Leftover slices hold together well after being refrigerated and are good
for lunch the next day.

PER SERVING: CALORIES 161; PROTEIN 6g; CARBOHYDRATES 23g; TOTAL FAT 6.1g; SATURATED FAT 0.6g; SODIUM 48mg; FIBER 4.6g; BETA-CAROTENE 756mcg; VITAMIN C 17mg; CALCIUM 40mg; IRON 1.8mg; FOLATE 116mcg; MAGNESIUM 49mg; ZINC 1.1mg; SELENIUM 6.1mcg

Agar is a vegan product produced from a variety of seaweeds. It's used as a stabilizing and thickening agent and is sold in health food stores and some supermarkets in both flake and powder forms. If using agar flakes instead of powder, double the amount.

BURGERS, PIZZA, AND FAST FOOD

Arugula- and Spinach-Stuffed Pitas with Watercress Pesto
Serves: 4

Pesto
- 1 bulb garlic
- 2 cups watercress, stems removed
- 5 leaves basil
- ½ cup walnuts
- 4 tablespoons unsweetened soy, hemp, or almond milk

Sandwich
- 4 pitas (100% whole grain)
- 1 tomato, sliced
- ½ cup thinly sliced red onion
- 2 cups arugula
- 2 cups spinach
- 1 avocado, pit removed, sliced

Roast garlic for 15 minutes at 300°F. Cut open cloves and squeeze out soft cooked garlic. Combine roasted garlic with other pesto ingredients in a high-powered blender and blend until smooth. Spread pesto on whole grain pitas. Stuff pita with remaining sandwich ingredients.

Non-vegan option: Add to each pita 1–2 ounces of oven-baked white-meat chicken or turkey, sliced or chopped.

PER SERVING: CALORIES 356; PROTEIN 11g; CARBOHYDRATES 43g; TOTAL FAT 17.3g; SATURATED FAT 2g; SODIUM 152mg; FIBER 6.6g; BETA-CAROTENE 1,653mcg; VITA-MIN C 22mg; CALCIUM 133mg; IRON 3.1mg; FOLATE 164mcg; MAGNESIUM 76mg; ZINC 1.5mg; SELENIUM 17.5mcg

Crispy Mushroom Fries
Serves: 2

½ cup raw almonds, toasted
1 tablespoon cornmeal
1 tablespoon nutritional yeast
2 teaspoons chia seeds
¼ teaspoon onion powder
¼ teaspoon garlic powder
⅛ teaspoon black pepper
2 large portobello mushrooms, gills removed, sliced
    ¼ inch thick
½ cup chickpea flour
1 cup no-salt-added or low-sodium vegetable broth

Preheat oven to 425°F. Place almonds in a food processor and pulse until chopped to the consistency of coarse bread crumbs. Remove from food processor, and in a shallow bowl combine with cornmeal, nutritional yeast, chia seeds, onion powder, garlic powder, and pepper.

Dredge portobello slices in chickpea flour; dip them in the vegetable broth and then into the almond mixture. Place on a baking sheet, lightly greased with olive oil, and bake for 10 minutes; turn and bake an additional 5–10 minutes, until golden brown.

Note: If desired, serve with no-salt-added or low-sodium marinara sauce for dipping.

PER SERVING: CALORIES 180; PROTEIN 9g; CARBOHYDRATES 20g; TOTAL FAT 8.2g; SATURATED FAT 0.7g; SODIUM 19mg; FIBER 6.6g; BETA-CAROTENE 7mcg; VITAMIN C 1mg; CALCIUM 71mg; IRON 3mg; FOLATE 215mcg; MAGNESIUM 72mg; ZINC 1.7mg; SELENIUM 11.2mcg

Easy Vegetable Pizza

Serves: 4

> 4 large pitas (100% whole grain)
> 2 cups no-salt-added or low-sodium pasta sauce
> ½ cup chopped shiitake mushrooms
> ½ cup chopped red onion
> 10 ounces frozen broccoli florets, thawed and finely chopped
> 2 ounces shredded nondairy mozzarella-type cheese

Preheat oven to 200°F. Place pitas on two baking sheets and warm
for 10 minutes. Remove from oven and spoon on the pasta sauce.
Sprinkle evenly with mushrooms, onion, and broccoli. Add a light
sprinkle of cheese. Bake for 30 minutes.

PER SERVING: CALORIES 229; PROTEIN 12g; CARBOHYDRATES 47g; TOTAL FAT 2.4g;
SATURATED FAT 0.3g; SODIUM 190mg; FIBER 9.7g; BETA-CAROTENE 686mcg; VITA-
MIN C 57mg; CALCIUM 165mg; IRON 2.7mg; FOLATE 67mcg; MAGNESIUM 83mg;
ZINC 1.9mg; SELENIUM 8.7mcg

Flax and Sesame Crackers

Serves: 8

> 1 cup ground flaxseeds
> ¼ cup unhulled sesame seeds
> ¼ cup coarsely chopped pumpkin seeds
> ¾ cup water, or more if needed
> ½ teaspoon garlic powder
> ½ teaspoon onion powder

Preheat oven to 350°F. Mix all ingredients in a mixing bowl until a dough forms, adding more water if needed. Spread evenly on parchment-lined baking sheet. Score into squares so they break evenly after baking. Bake for 30–35 minutes or until crisp and lightly browned.

Makes about 16 crackers.

Note: You can substitute a variety of seasonings for, or use in addition to, the onion and garlic powder. Try fresh or dried herbs, chili powder, nutritional yeast, Dr. Fuhrman's MatoZest, cinnamon, chopped dates, or raisins.

PER SERVING: CALORIES 55; PROTEIN 2g; CARBOHYDRATES 3g; TOTAL FAT 4.5g; SATURATED FAT 0.6g; SODIUM 2mg; FIBER 1.9g; BETA-CAROTENE 7mcg; CALCIUM 33mg; IRON 1mg; FOLATE 8mcg; MAGNESIUM 44mg; ZINC 0.6mg; SELENIUM 1.7mcg

Kale Chips
Serves: 3

> 1 bunch kale, tough stems and center ribs removed
> Half olive oil and half water mixture in a spray bottle

Choice of Seasonings:
> Garlic and/or onion powder
> Balsamic vinegar
> Fresh lemon juice
> Dr. Fuhrman's VegiZest or MatoZest, Mrs. Dash seasoning blend,
>   or no-salt Spike
> Nutritional yeast
> Chili powder
> Black pepper
> Raw cashew or almond butter mixed with water

Preheat oven to 225°F. Tear kale into uniform, chip-size pieces. Spread evenly on a nonstick baking sheet. Shake olive oil and water mixture well and spray kale lightly. Sprinkle with your choice of seasoning. Bake for 50 minutes, or until crispy and dry, tossing occasionally to prevent burning. Eat as a snack or use as a topping for salads or other dishes.

PER SERVING: CALORIES 123; PROTEIN 4g; CARBOHYDRATES 8g; TOTAL FAT 9.6g; SATURATED FAT 0.9g; SODIUM 22mg; FIBER 1.5g; BETA-CAROTENE 4,359mcg; VITAMIN C 57mg; CALCIUM 106mg; IRON 1.4mg; FOLATE 24mcg; MAGNESIUM 63mg; ZINC 0.7mg; SELENIUM 0.4mcg

Bean Burger Tips

Bean burgers are great because you probably have the ingredients on hand to make a batch at any given time. They work for a quick evening meal, and leftovers can be packed for lunch the next day. You can make them regular burger size or make smaller patties for bean burger sliders. Bean burger variations are endless, but my basic formula consists of beans, a source of fat such as seeds or nuts, a grain, and some veggies and flavoring ingredients. For example, my simple Sunny Bean Burgers contain just six ingredients: kidney or pinto beans, sunflower seeds, oats, minced onion, low-sodium ketchup, and a dash of chili powder.

Bean Burger Ingredients

Beans: You can use any variety of cooked, canned, or boxed beans—black, red kidney, pinto, or white beans; lentils or chickpeas. Mash them up well.

Nut and Seeds: Ground or chopped nuts and/or seeds provide the healthy fat.

Grains: Grains help to bind the other ingredients together. Oats are a common ingredient in bean burgers, but you can also use cooked rice, cooked quinoa, or a small amount of whole grain bread crumbs.

Vegetables: Diced mushrooms are great in burgers. In addition to adding a meaty texture, they provide *umami,* or the fifth taste in addition to sweet, salty, sour, and bitter. Umami is defined as robust, savory, and meaty. You can also add shredded carrots, chopped spinach, chopped kale, diced artichoke, or mashed sweet potato.

Onions and Garlic: Onions and garlic give a flavor boost without added salt. They are also in the *Allium* genus of vegetables, which have beneficial effects on the cardiovascular and immune systems.

Tempeh: Tempeh is made from cooked and slightly fermented soybeans that are formed into a firm patty. It provides an interesting flavor and chewiness and can be grated or crumbled and added to burgers.

Tofu: Freeze extra firm tofu, defrost it, squeeze out the excess moisture, and then crumble and add it to burgers for a light but chewy texture.

continued

For Meat Lovers: You don't really need meat since bean burgers taste so good, but if you want them to taste meaty, add 1 ounce of ground organic/wild meat or fowl per person for a burger that tastes even better than traditional all-beef patties.

Toppings: Add sliced red onion, sliced tomato, lettuce, avocado, sautéed mushrooms, and/or low-sodium/no-corn-syrup ketchup.

Bread: If desired, serve burgers on a small pita, half a roll, or a slice of bread. Make sure your bread choices are 100% whole grain. See page 271 for more advice on choosing bread products.

Sunny Bean Burgers
Serves: 2

> ¼ cup sunflower seeds
> 2 cups cooked kidney or pinto beans, or canned no-salt-added or
>   low-sodium kidney or pinto beans, drained
> ½ cup minced onion
> 2 tablespoons low-sodium ketchup
> 1 tablespoon old-fashioned rolled oats
> ½ teaspoon chili powder

Preheat oven to 350°F. Lightly oil a baking sheet with a little olive oil on a paper towel. Chop sunflower seeds in a food processor or with a hand chopper. Mash beans in the food processor or with a potato masher and mix with the sunflower seeds. Mix in remaining ingredients and form into six patties.

Place patties on the baking sheet and bake for 25 minutes. Remove from the oven and let cool slightly, until you can pick up each patty and compress it firmly in your hands to reform the burger. Return the patties to the baking sheet, bottom side up, and bake for another 10 minutes.

Note: If desired, you can cook these on a grill.

PER SERVING: CALORIES 369; PROTEIN 21g; CARBOHYDRATES 53g; TOTAL FAT 10.2g; SATURATED FAT 1.1g; SODIUM 13mg; FIBER 14.4g; BETA-CAROTENE 187mcg; VITAMIN C 8mg; CALCIUM 97mg; IRON 5.5mg; FOLATE 282mcg; MAGNESIUM 153mg; ZINC 2.9mg; SELENIUM 13.8mcg

White Bean, Wild Rice, and Almond Burgers

Serves: 10

½ cup uncooked wild rice, rinsed
1 cup finely chopped red onions
1 cup finely chopped celery
3 cloves garlic, minced
¼ teaspoon dried basil
¼ teaspoon dried parsley
¼ teaspoon Mrs. Dash Original no-salt seasoning blend
½ cup raw almonds, lightly toasted
1½ cups cooked white beans, or 1 (15-ounce) can no-salt-added
   or low-sodium white beans, drained
Bread crumbs (100% whole grain), or old-fashioned oats, if
   needed to adjust consistency

Combine rice and 2 cups water (or no-salt-added or low-sodium vegetable broth for additional flavor) in a saucepan. Bring to a boil, reduce heat, cover, and simmer for 45 minutes or until rice is tender. Drain any excess water.

While rice is cooking, water-sauté onions, celery, and garlic over low flame for 10 minutes, or until tender. Stir frequently to prevent burning; cover sporadically to soften vegetables, but uncover to let water steam off. Stir in basil, parsley, and Mrs. Dash.

Finely chop almonds in food processor. Add beans and process until beans are pureed and mixture is well combined. Place in a bowl and stir in wild rice and onion mixture. Form into burgers. If mixture is too wet, add a small amount of whole grain bread crumbs or oats. Place burgers on a baking sheet lined with parchment paper. Bake at 350°F for 40 minutes, turning after 20 minutes.

PER SERVING: CALORIES 117; PROTEIN 6g; CARBOHYDRATES 16g; TOTAL FAT 3.9g; SATURATED FAT 0.3g; SODIUM 13mg; FIBER 3.4g; BETA-CAROTENE 29mcg; VITAMIN C 2mg; CALCIUM 51mg; IRON 1.5mg; FOLATE 38mcg; MAGNESIUM 54mg; ZINC 1.1mg; SELENIUM 1mcg

CHOOSE ORGANIC MEATS

If you choose to include a small amount of meat in your diet, select certified organic products. You can be sure that the animal feed is grown without chemical pesticides and the animal is not treated with antibiotics or hormones. The animals also must have access to outdoor exercise areas, sunlight, and pasture. Organic farms are monitored, and the producers are held responsible for their practices. "Natural" meats may follow some or all of the organic practices, but they don't have to. "Natural" as well as "grass fed" are voluntary terms and aren't monitored. They can refer to a wide range of practices.

Meat-Lover's Beef, Bean, and Mushroom Burgers

Serves: 7

1 small onion, chopped
1 clove garlic, minced
2 cups mushrooms, chopped
¼ cup unhulled sesame seeds
1½ cups cooked red kidney beans, or 1 (15-ounce) can no-salt-
   added or low-sodium kidney beans, drained
1 teaspoon dry basil
½ teaspoon dry oregano
⅛ teaspoon black pepper
1 cup cooked black rice
6 ounces (about 1 cup) organic ground beef (see Note for
   vegan option)

Preheat oven to 300°F. Water-sauté onions and garlic until they begin to soften, about 2 minutes. Add mushrooms and cook for about 5 minutes, until all liquid is evaporated.

Grind sesame seeds in food processor. Add mushroom mixture, beans, and spices and process until well combined. Spoon into a bowl and mix in cooked black rice and beef.

Form into 7 medium-size patties. Place burgers on a baking sheet lined with parchment paper or lightly wiped with olive oil. Bake for 40 minutes, turning after 20 minutes.

Note: To make without ground beef, use an additional 1½ cups cooked beans.

PER SERVING: CALORIES 238; PROTEIN 12g; CARBOHYDRATES 32g; TOTAL FAT 7.1g; SATURATED FAT 1.8g; CHOLESTEROL 16.5mg; SODIUM 20mg; FIBER 4.2g; BETA-CAROTENE 16mcg; VITAMIN C 3mg; CALCIUM 81mg; IRON 3.8mg; FOLATE 64mcg; MAGNESIUM 45mg; ZINC 2.1mg; SELENIUM 7.3mcg

Black Bean and Turkey Burgers

Serves: 7

>   2 cups chopped mushrooms
>   ½ cup old-fashioned rolled oats
>   ¼ cup raw pumpkin seeds
>   2 carrots, grated
>   1½ cups cooked black beans, or 1 (15-ounce) can low-sodium
>   or no-salt-added black beans, drained
>   ½ teaspoon cumin
>   ½ teaspoon coriander
>   ½ teaspoon chili powder
>   ½ teaspoon onion powder
>   ¼ teaspoon black pepper
>   ⅛ teaspoon cayenne pepper
>   6 ounces (about 1 cup) ground organic turkey (see Note for
>   vegan option)

Preheat oven to 300°F. Heat 1–2 tablespoons water in a small pan and sauté mushrooms until tender and moisture has evaporated, about 5 minutes. Set aside.

Grind oats and pumpkin seeds in a food processor. Add grated carrots, three-quarters of the beans, and all of the spices and process until blended. Spoon mixture into a mixing bowl and mix in sautéed mushrooms, remaining whole beans, and ground turkey.

Form into 7 medium-size patties. Place burgers on a baking sheet lined with parchment paper or lightly wiped with olive oil. Bake for 40 minutes, turning once after 20 minutes.

Note: To make without ground turkey, use an additional 1½ cups cooked beans.

PER SERVING: CALORIES 148; PROTEIN 11g; CARBOHYDRATES 16g; TOTAL FAT 5.1g; SATURATED FAT 1.1g; CHOLESTEROL 19.2mg; SODIUM 40mg; FIBER 4.9g; BETA-CAROTENE 1,491mcg; VITAMIN C 2mg; CALCIUM 25mg; IRON 2.3mg; FOLATE 70mcg; MAGNESIUM 77mg; ZINC 1.6mg; SELENIUM 9.8mcg

Tofu Fingers Marinara

Serves: 6

1 block extra firm tofu, drained
1 cup raw almonds, toasted
2 tablespoons cornmeal
2 tablespoons nutritional yeast
¼ teaspoon garlic powder
¼ teaspoon dried basil
¼ teaspoon dried oregano
⅛ teaspoon cayenne pepper, or to taste
1 cup no-salt-added or low-sodium marinara sauce, divided

Preheat oven to 375°F. Wrap tofu in several layers of paper towels and place on a plate or cutting board. Cover with a second plate and balance a heavy can or two on top to weigh down the plate and press the tofu. Set aside and let drain for 30 minutes. Remove and discard paper towels. Slice the tofu into ½-inch-thick slices.

Place almonds in food processor and pulse until chopped to the consistency of coarse bread crumbs. Remove from food processor and combine with cornmeal, nutritional yeast, garlic powder, basil, oregano, and cayenne pepper.

Place ½ cup marinara sauce in a bowl. Dip the tofu pieces into the marinara and then place them in the almond mixture, pressing lightly to cover both sides well. Gently shake off any excess nut mixture. Lay flat on a baking sheet. Bake, flipping every 10–15 minutes, for 40–45 minutes. Serve with remaining marinara sauce for dipping.

PER SERVING: CALORIES 282; PROTEIN 15g; CARBOHYDRATES 17g; TOTAL FAT 18.1g; SATURATED FAT 1.7g; SODIUM 23mg; FIBER 5.7g; BETA-CAROTENE 163mcg; VITA-MIN C 5mg; CALCIUM 128mg; IRON 2.8mg; FOLATE 123mcg; MAGNESIUM 159mg; ZINC 1.1mg; SELENIUM 1.5mcg

Zucchini Bean Burrito

Serves: 6

    1 red onion, chopped
    2 cloves garlic, chopped
    1 green poblano chili pepper, seeded and thinly sliced
    1 medium tomato, chopped
    2 cups zucchini, chopped
    3 cups cooked pinto beans, or 2 (15-ounce) cans low-sodium
        or no-salt-added pinto beans, drained
    1 tablespoon chili powder
    1 teaspoon ground cumin
    2 tablespoons chopped cilantro
    6 large (100% whole grain) tortillas
    3 cups shredded romaine lettuce or mixed greens
    1 ripe avocado, sliced
    1 cup low-sodium or no-salt-added salsa

Heat 2 tablespoons water in a large skillet. Add onion, garlic, and poblano chili pepper and water-sauté until tender, about 3 minutes. Add tomato and zucchini; continue cooking for an additional 5 minutes or until zucchini is soft. Add beans, chili powder, and cumin; stir to combine and cook for 10 minutes.

Using a potato masher or back of a spoon, thoroughly mash bean mixture. Stir in cilantro. Spread beans on tortillas, top with lettuce, avocado, and salsa and roll up. Beans may also be served as a side dish or dip.

PER SERVING: CALORIES 361; PROTEIN 18g; CARBOHYDRATES 73g; TOTAL FAT 10.7g; SATURATED FAT 2.1g; SODIUM 126mg; FIBER 14.6g; BETA-CAROTENE 1,603mcg; VITAMIN C 77mg; CALCIUM 109mg; IRON 5.6mg; FOLATE 326mcg; MAGNESIUM 94mg; ZINC 1.9mg; SELENIUM 22.8mcg

Healthy Bread Choices

If you choose to eat bread, don't make your decision on the basis of claims made on the front of the package. You need to learn about the different options and look at the fine print on the list of ingredients.

Whole Grain Bread: "Whole grain" means that all parts of the grain are still present. A whole grain has three components:

Germ: The embryo or sprouting section of the seed.

Endosperm: The bulk of the interior of the seed.

Bran: The outer layer that holds everything together.

When wheat is refined to make white flour, the bran and germ are stripped away, along with most of the nutrients, leaving only the endosperm, which is ground into flour. Look for breads that contain only 100 percent whole grains. Breads that are made with whole grains that are more coarsely ground are the healthiest choice. The more finely ground the grain, such as whole wheat pastry flour, the higher the glycemic load. Breads that are labeled "made with whole grains" often contain some whole grain but include refined flour as well. In addition to wheat, whole grain products can be made with barley, millet, rye, brown rice, and oats. Intact whole grains have not been ground into flour and are usually eaten after being softened by boiling.

Sprouted Grain Bread: Sprouted grain breads are made from whole wheat kernels or other whole grains that are allowed to sprout and then are ground up. As far as nutrition goes, they are the best whole grain choice.

Whole wheat bread: Whole wheat bread is a type of whole grain bread made from whole wheat flour. Look for bread made from 100 percent whole wheat flour. This should be the first ingredient listed and the only flour mentioned in the ingredients. Many products claiming to be "whole wheat" are simply white bread with a little extra whole wheat flour added, along with some food coloring.

Multigrain and Seeded Breads: Breads containing mixed grains and seeds can appear to be healthful, but many of them fall short when compared with

100 percent whole wheat or 100 percent whole grain breads. Some consist mainly of processed white flour, with grains and seeds making up only a small proportion of the ingredients. A "multigrain" label only tells you that the bread contains different kinds of grains; it doesn't mean they haven't been refined.

White Bread: You should avoid white bread because it lacks the nutrients contained in less processed grain products. Some labeling terms can be misleading and make products appear healthful. The terms "wheat flour"; "unbleached wheat flour"; "enriched wheat flour"; "stone-ground wheat flour"; "multigrain," "five grain," or "seven grain"; and "100 percent wheat flour or bran" are all sometimes merely a way of saying "refined white flour." Wheat flour is just another name for white flour. Any time you see "enriched," you know that you're getting white flour. Flour that has been refined and stripped of its bran and germ must have some of the B vitamins and iron replaced by enrichment.

In addition to the form of grain used in a bread product, watch out for unhealthy fats. Don't choose a product that contains hydrogenated vegetable oil, *trans* fats, partially hydrogenated oil, or vegetable oil shortening. Also avoid products containing high-fructose corn syrup or a high level of sodium. A slice of bread should contain no more than 180 milligrams of sodium per slice and should provide at least 3 grams of fiber.

Table 18 lists some bread products that I recommend.

TABLE 18. RECOMMENDED BREAD PRODUCTS

BRAND	PRODUCT	SODIUM (mg per slice or piece)	FIBER (g per slice or piece)	INGREDIENT NOTES
Food for Life	7 Sprouted Grains Bread	80	3	Sprouted wheat, rye, barley, oats, millet, corn, and brown rice
Food for Life	Bran for Life Bread	140	5	100% whole wheat flour
Food for Life	Ezekiel 4:9 Sprouted Whole Grain Bread	75	3	Sprouted wheat, barley, millet, lentils, soybeans, spelt
Food for Life	Ezekiel 4:9 Whole Grain Pocket Bread	110	3	100% whole wheat flour
Food for Life	Ezekiel 4:9 Sprouted Whole Grain Tortillas	140	5	Sprouted wheat, soybeans, barley, millet, lentils, and spelt
Manna Organics	Multigrain	10	4	Sprouted wheat, brown rice, barley, oats, millet, rye
Manna Organics	Sunseed	3	7	Sprouted wheat; sunflower, sesame, flax, poppy, and caraway seeds
Manna Organics	Fruit & Nut	7	6	Sprouted wheat, raisins, dates, almonds, cashews, hazelnuts
Alvarado Street Bakery	Sprouted Wheat Multi-Grain	170	2	Sprouted wheat, millet, corn, rye, sunflower seeds
Alvarado Street Bakery	Sprouted Whole Wheat	180	2	Sprouted wheat, dates, raisins
Alvarado Street Bakery	No Salt Sprouted Multi-Grain	10	2	Sprouted wheat, millet, corn, rye, sunflower seeds
Pepperidge Farm	100% Natural Whole Wheat	130	3	Whole wheat flour; contains sugar and oil
Natural Ovens Bakery	Whole Grain Naturals	130	4	Whole wheat flour; contains sugar and oil

DESSERTS

Apple Surprise

Serves: 6

> 1 cup raisins
> ¼ cup water
> 8 apples, peeled, cored, and diced
> ½ cup chopped walnuts
> 4 tablespoons ground flaxseeds
> 1 tablespoon cinnamon

Place raisins in a pot and cover with ¼ cup water. Place diced apples on top. Cover and simmer to steam the apples over very low heat for 7 minutes. Transfer apple/raisin mixture to a bowl and mix well with remaining ingredients.

Note: This recipe keeps well in the refrigerator for 7 days.

PER SERVING: CALORIES 260; PROTEIN 7g; CARBOHYDRATES 48g; TOTAL FAT 8.8g; SATURATED FAT 0.8g; SODIUM 7mg; FIBER 7.9g; BETA-CAROTENE 51mcg; VITAMIN C 10mg; CALCIUM 59mg; IRON 1.7mg; FOLATE 21mcg; MAGNESIUM 51mg; ZINC 0.7mg; SELENIUM 1.8mcg

Banana Mango Sorbet
Serves: 2

    1 ripe banana, frozen
    2 cups frozen mango
    4 slices unsweetened dried mango
    ¼ cup almond, hemp, or soy milk
    6 ice cubes

Add all ingredients to a high-powered blender and blend until smooth and creamy.

Note: You can substitute 4 Medjool or 8 Deglet Noor dates for the dried mango.

PER SERVING: CALORIES 308; PROTEIN 4g; CARBOHYDRATES 79g; TOTAL FAT 1.3g; SATURATED FAT 0.2g; SODIUM 21mg; FIBER 8.1g; BETA-CAROTENE 902mcg; VITAMIN C 51mg; CALCIUM 62mg; IRON 1.1mg; FOLATE 47mcg; MAGNESIUM 64mg; ZINC 0.5mg; SELENIUM 3.0mcg

BE READY WITH FROZEN BANANAS
Bananas are a great ingredient for a number of desserts. Peel ripe bananas and wrap them tightly in plastic wrap or place in a plastic bag. Freeze at least 12 hours before you want to use them.

Black Cherry Sorbet

Serves: 3

3 cups frozen sweet black cherries
1 cup vanilla soy, hemp, or almond milk
1 ripe banana, frozen
½ cup walnuts
3 Medjool or 6 Deglet Noor dates, pitted

Blend all ingredients in a high-powered blender.

PER SERVING: CALORIES 249; PROTEIN 6g; CARBOHYDRATES 37g; TOTAL FAT 11g; SATURATED FAT 1.1g; SODIUM 34mg; FIBER 5.3g; BETA-CAROTENE 273mcg; VITAMIN C 8mg; CALCIUM 60mg; IRON 1.6mg; FOLATE 35mcg; MAGNESIUM 64mg; ZINC 0.9mg; SELENIUM 3.9mcg

THE SECRET TO MAKING EASY AND DELICIOUS SORBETS AND THICK SHAKES

Blend together one bag of frozen fruit with one fresh fruit and a little nondairy milk. To make a creamy ice cream instead of a sorbet, add a healthy fat source such as hulled hemp seeds, cashews, coconut flakes, or macadamia nuts. Frozen desserts that contain some fat from nuts or seeds will stay softer and can be stored in the freezer before serving.

Blueberry Banana Cobbler
Serves: 2

1 banana, sliced
1 cup frozen blueberries
¼ cup old-fashioned rolled oats
1 tablespoon dried currants
¼ vanilla bean, or ¼ teaspoon alcohol-free vanilla extract
2 tablespoons chopped raw almonds
2 tablespoons unsweetened, shredded coconut
¼ teaspoon cinnamon

Combine banana, berries, oats, currants, and vanilla in a microwave-safe dish. If using a vanilla bean, scrape pulp and seeds from bean with a dull knife and add them to the mix; discard pod. Microwave for 2 minutes. Top with almonds, coconut, and cinnamon and microwave for 1 minute. Serve warm.

PER SERVING: CALORIES 195; PROTEIN 3g; CARBOHYDRATES 35g; TOTAL FAT 6g; SATURATED FAT 1.9g; SODIUM 3mg; FIBER 6.2g; BETA-CAROTENE 39mcg; VITAMIN C 8mg; CALCIUM 32mg; IRON 1.4mg; FOLATE 25mcg; MAGNESIUM 66mg; ZINC 0.7mg; SELENIUM 4.8mcg

Chunky Blueberry Walnut Sorbet

Serves: 4

1¼ cups unsweetened soy, hemp, or almond milk (use 1 cup for
thicker sorbet and 1½ cups for thinner sorbet)
3 cups frozen blueberries, divided
2 ripe bananas, frozen, one chopped into bite-size pieces
¾ cup chopped walnuts, divided
1 tablespoon ground flaxseeds

Blend nondairy milk, 2 cups frozen blueberries, 1 frozen banana
(unchopped), and ½ cup walnuts in high-powered blender. Empty
into a chilled bowl and mix in remaining blueberries, chopped
banana, and remaining walnuts. Serve topped with ground flaxseeds.

PER SERVING: CALORIES 303; PROTEIN 8g; CARBOHYDRATES 35g; TOTAL FAT 17.4g;
SATURATED FAT 1.7g; SODIUM 44mg; FIBER 7.5g; BETA-CAROTENE 326mcg; VITA-
MIN C 8mg; CALCIUM 67mg; IRON 1.9mg; FOLATE 55mcg; MAGNESIUM 82mg; ZINC
1.3mg; SELENIUM 5.8mcg

Cocoa Ice Bean

Serves: 4

2 ripe bananas, frozen
½ cup raw cashews
¾ cup cooked black beans, or canned no-salt-added or low-sodium black beans, drained
3 tablespoons natural nonalkalized cocoa powder
5 Medjool dates or 10 Deglet Noor dates, pitted
½ vanilla bean, split lengthwise, or ½ teaspoon alcohol-free vanilla extract
1 cup soy, hemp, or almond milk

Blend all ingredients together in a high-powered blender until very smooth. If using a vanilla bean, scrape pulp and seeds from pod with a dull knife and add them to blender; discard pod. Add additional nondairy milk if needed to adjust consistency. Pour into bowl and freeze until firm. Allow to soften slightly before serving.

PER SERVING: CALORIES 254; PROTEIN 10g; CARBOHYDRATES 38g; TOTAL FAT 9.5g; SATURATED FAT 1.9g; SODIUM 37mg; FIBER 7.6g; BETA-CAROTENE 236mcg; VITAMIN C 5mg; CALCIUM 49mg; IRON 3.2mg; FOLATE 76mcg; MAGNESIUM 125mg; ZINC 2mg; SELENIUM 8mcg

Medjool dates are larger and sweeter than the more common Deglet Noor date. In recipes that call for dates, substitute 2 Deglet Noor dates for 1 Medjool.

Fudgy Black Bean Brownies

Serves: 12

> 2 cups cooked black beans or canned no-salt-added or low-
> sodium black beans, drained
> 10 Medjool or 20 Deglet Noor dates, pitted
> 2 tablespoons raw almond butter
> ½ vanilla bean, or ½ teaspoon alcohol-free vanilla extract
> ½ cup natural nonalkalized cocoa powder
> 1 tablespoon ground chia seeds

Preheat oven to 200°F. Combine black beans, dates, almond butter, and vanilla in a food processor or high-powered blender. If using a vanilla bean, scrape pulp and seeds from pod with a dull knife and add them to blender; discard pod. Blend until smooth. Add cocoa powder and chia seeds and blend again.

Spread into a very lightly oiled 8-by-8-inch baking pan. Bake for 1½ hours. Cool completely and apply topping if desired. Cut into small squares. Store in a covered container in the refrigerator for up to one week.

Optional Topping

> 1 ripe avocado
> ½ cup water
> 4 tablespoons natural nonalkalized cocoa powder
> 5 Medjool dates, pitted

Blend topping ingredients in a high-powered blender.

PER SERVING: CALORIES 125; PROTEIN 4g; CARBOHYDRATES 25g; TOTAL FAT 2g; SAT-URATED FAT 0.5g; SODIUM 2mg; FIBER 5.6g; BETA-CAROTENE 18mcg; CALCIUM 40mg; IRON 1.5mg; FOLATE 50mcg; MAGNESIUM 58mg; ZINC 0.8mg; SELENIUM 0.9mcg

> Agar is a vegetarian gelatin made from seaweed that you can use as a thickening agent in a variety of recipes. It's available at many health food stores and in some supermarkets. If using agar flakes instead of powder, double the amount.

Oatmeal Raisin Cookies Filled with Blueberry Jam

Serves: 14

1½ cups blueberries

1 cup red or black grapes

½ teaspoon agar powder (see Box on page 280)

2 teaspoons arrowroot

2 ripe bananas, mashed (add extra banana if batter is too dry)

1½ cups old-fashioned rolled oats

½ cup raisins, soaked in water for 30 minutes, then drained

⅓ cup chopped almonds or walnuts

¼ cup unsweetened, shredded coconut

½ vanilla bean, split lengthwise, or ½ teaspoon alcohol-free
vanilla extract

⅛ teaspoon cinnamon

To make the blueberry jam:

Combine blueberries, grapes, agar powder, and arrowroot in a high-powered blender. Transfer to a small saucepan and slowly bring to a boil over medium heat, stirring occasionally. Boil for 2 minutes (but no longer), stirring constantly. Remove from heat and allow to cool. Place in covered container and refrigerate until ready to use. Makes 2 cups.

To make the cookies:

Preheat oven to 325°F. Combine mashed banana and oats. Add soaked raisins, nuts, coconut, vanilla, and cinnamon. If using a vanilla bean, scrape pulp and seeds from pod with a dull knife and add them to mixture; discard pod. Mix well.

Drop by tablespoons onto a nonstick cookie sheet. Flatten a little, make an indentation in the center of the cookie, and add blueberry jam in the indentation. Bake for 13 minutes, or until golden. Makes 14 cookies.

ONE COOKIE: CALORIES 98; PROTEIN 4g; CARBOHYDRATES 19g; TOTAL FAT 2.4g; SATURATED FAT 0.6g; SODIUM 2mg; FIBER 2.4g; BETA-CAROTENE 14mcg; VITAMIN C 4mg; CALCIUM 11mg; IRON 0.8mg; FOLATE 10mcg; MAGNESIUM 38mg; ZINC 0.4mg; SELENIUM 3.3mcg

Strawberry Panna Cotta

Serves: 4

For the Panna Cotta:
 2 cups frozen strawberries
 2 cups soy, hemp, or almond milk
 3 Medjool or 6 Deglet Noor dates, pitted
 ½ vanilla bean, split lengthwise, or 1 teaspoon alcohol-free
  vanilla extract
 1 tablespoon agar powder (see Note)

For the Sauce:
 1½ cups frozen strawberries
 ½ cup soy, hemp, or almond milk
 3 Medjool or 6 Deglet Noor dates, pitted
 ¼ cup raw cashews

Blend strawberries, nondairy milk, and dates in a high-powered blender until smooth. Add blended mixture to a medium saucepan. If using a vanilla bean, scrape pulp and seeds from the pod with a dull knife. Add pulp, seeds, and pod to the saucepan along with the agar powder. Cook over medium heat until mixture starts to boil. Reduce heat to low and simmer for 5 minutes, stirring constantly. Remove vanilla pod.

Pour into 4 glasses or small bowls. Refrigerate overnight. It should be firm.

To make the sauce, blend frozen strawberries, nondairy milk, dates, and cashews in a high-powered blender until smooth. To serve, spoon some of the berry sauce on top of each panna cotta.

Note: If using agar flakes instead of powder, double the amount.

PER SERVING: CALORIES 297; PROTEIN 9g; CARBOHYDRATES 54g; TOTAL FAT 7.5g; SATURATED FAT 1.1g; SODIUM 85mg; FIBER 8.3g; BETA-CAROTENE 621mcg; VITAMIN C 3mg; CALCIUM 95mg; IRON 2.8mg; FOLATE 42mcg; MAGNESIUM 90mg; ZINC 1.4mg; SELENIUM 9mcg

Summer Fruit Pie

Serves: 8

For Pie Shell:
  1 cup almonds
  1 cup dates, pitted (Medjool, if available)
  2 tablespoons unsweetened shredded coconut

For Pie Filling:
  2–3 bananas, sliced
  1 teaspoon lemon juice
  2 kiwis, sliced
  1 quart organic strawberries, sliced
  1 pint blueberries
  ½ cup vanilla soy, hemp, or almond milk
  1¼ cups frozen strawberries, or 1 pint fresh organic strawberries
  2 dates, pitted

Make pie shell by placing almonds in a food processor or high-powered blender and processing until very fine. Add dates and process until chopped and mixed well. Remove from food processor and knead shredded coconut in by hand. Add a small amount of water if needed to hold mixture together. Press into 9-inch pie plate to form shell.

To make the filling, spread bananas on the crust, pressing down slightly. Sprinkle lemon juice over bananas. Place kiwis, strawberries, and blueberries over bananas. If desired, reserve some fruit to decorate top of pie.

Add nondairy milk, frozen strawberries, and dates in a blender and blend until smooth. Pour blended mixture over the fruit. Decorate with additional fruit as desired. Cover and freeze for at least 2 hours before serving.

PER SERVING: CALORIES 245; PROTEIN 9g; CARBOHYDRATES 47g; TOTAL FAT 6.8g; SATURATED FAT 0.6g; SODIUM 11mg; FIBER 8g; BETA-CAROTENE 101mcg; VITAMIN C 76mg; CALCIUM 70mg; IRON 1.6mg; FOLATE 47mcg; MAGNESIUM 75mg; ZINC 0.8mg; SELENIUM 2.7mcg

Vanilla Coconut Nice Cream

Serves: 4

> 20 walnut halves
> ½ vanilla bean, split lengthwise, or 1 tablespoon alcohol-free
>   vanilla extract
> 4 medium bananas, frozen
> ½ cup unsweetened creamed coconut (see Note)
> ¼ cup soy, hemp, or almond milk

Using a high-powered blender, blend walnuts on high speed until the consistency of dust. If using a vanilla bean, scrape pulp and seeds from pod with a dull knife and add them to the blender along with remaining ingredients (discard vanilla bean pod). Blend on very high speed until silky smooth. Serve immediately, or store in freezer for later use.

Note: Creamed coconut is unsweetened dehydrated coconut meat ground to a semisolid creamy paste.

PER SERVING: CALORIES 292; PROTEIN 3g; CARBOHYDRATES 33g; TOTAL FAT 18.3g; SATURATED FAT 13.5g; SODIUM 10mg; FIBER 3.4g; BETA-CAROTENE 31mcg; VITAMIN C 11mg; CALCIUM 17mg; IRON 1.2mg; FOLATE 30mcg; MAGNESIUM 60mg; ZINC 0.8mg; SELENIUM 1.4mcg

Vanilla Cream Topping for Fruit

Serves: 8

   1 vanilla bean, split lengthwise, or 1 teaspoon alcohol-free
      vanilla extract
   1⅓ cups raw macadamia or cashew nuts
   1 cup soy, hemp, or almond milk
   ⅔ cup dates, pitted

If using vanilla bean, scrape pulp and seeds from pod with a dull knife; discard pod. Blend vanilla pulp and seeds, nuts, nondairy milk, and dates together in a high-powered blender until smooth and creamy. Serve over strawberries, other berries, or fruit. May also be used as a topping for fruit sorbets or baked desserts.

Note: For a Chocolate Cream Topping, add 2 tablespoons of natural nonalkalized cocoa powder.

PER SERVING: CALORIES 184; PROTEIN 6g; CARBOHYDRATES 20g; TOTAL FAT 10.7g; SATURATED FAT 1.9g; SODIUM 20mg; FIBER 2.3g; BETA-CAROTENE 111mcg; CALCIUM 26mg; IRON 2mg; FOLATE 13mcg; MAGNESIUM 81mg; ZINC 1.5mg; SELENIUM 6.4mcg

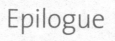

Epilogue

If you've come this far, you have demonstrated a respectable interest in nutritional science. Nutritional science is interesting and fun, because we can take what we've learned and put it into action every day, thereby taking control of our own health and fate. Nothing in life is more powerful than driving your own vehicle.

Despite diverse dietary beliefs, dietary camps, and the popularity of fad diets that come and go, sufficient scientific evidence exists to show us what the most healthful, weight-optimizing, and life-extending diet style should be. We have sufficient data, coupled with clinical experience, to take life-extending and life-saving actions with a strong degree of certainty. With time, as more and more science adds to this body of evidence, these same principles will remain irrefutable. In other words, superior nutrition can never go out of style, and further science will only support this information more and more—not change it in any significant way.

Some people—with their diverse motivations, beliefs, and preferences—may object to and fight the reality of this science-based nutritional guidance. *I don't want to eat like that. I can't eat like that. I would rather be dead than eat like that.* The nay-sayers are typically food addicts fighting to maintain their addictions with the "myth of moderation." Unfortunately, these are the same people who most need change, the same people who are so helplessly addicted that they can't even think about giving up their toxic and dangerous food habits, no matter how convincing or important the evidence.

What people claim they prefer or can or cannot do is irrelevant. People like what they are used to; change produces anxiety. The addicted mind sets up a whole series of rationalizations and excuses to avoid conflict. Nevertheless, nutritional science is not a popularity contest. The information should not be muddled and watered down to meet the objections of those people who seek mediocrity. Science continues to march forward, leaving behind those entrenched in conventional, established thinking and beliefs. The facts are that all people can follow this nutritarian diet style, and they can enjoy it immensely.

However, that enjoyment comes only to people who stick with it long enough to allow their taste preferences to change.

So, should you follow a nutritarian diet style 80 percent, 90 percent, or 100 percent? Certainly, you're behind the wheel, and how you steer is entirely up to you, but what I and many other long-time nutritarians have found is that we don't feel well after we eat second-class foods. Nor do we like them as much as we did in the past, because our tastes have changed. We simply choose not to eat them because we prefer healthier foods and recipes made in a healthier way. The miraculous benefits come predictably to those who maintain superior nutrition. It will take strength, it will take effort, but the pleasure and rewards you will get from a healthy life will be priceless.

Keeping yourself healthy so you can avoid needless medical care is one of the most important things you can do to improve the quality of your life. When you don't eat healthfully, you don't just shorten your life, you live a more troubled, sickly, and unhappy life. You can't enjoy living if you don't feel well and are sick all the time.

When you eat a nutritarian diet, on the other hand, you can enjoy eating more, because you don't have to skimp and eat thimble-size portions of food. You don't have to count calories, measure portions, or restrict eating healthy foods you enjoy. A nutritarian diet is focused on eating larger meals with more food volume.

And when you get yourself free of the pleasure trap set by super-stimulating junk foods and salt, your taste buds return to normal, which makes foods that promote health taste awesome.

Regardless of the economic power of the food, medical, and drug industries; regardless of the pressures of societal norms; regardless of the special interests trying to use questionable and distorted data to justify their preferences and influence government, nutritional science marches forward and will not be swayed.

Remember that excellent health also involves sufficient sleep, rest, recreation, and intellectual pursuits; healthy interpersonal relations;

exercise; and satisfaction in your personal accomplishments. When you strive to have a kind and positive effect on those whom your life touches, you will experience profound positive effects on your well-being—like eating wild berries and kale. Living isn't all about food, though food is our body's largest physical interaction with our external environment and affects all aspects of our lives.

Time and time again in my medical practice, I see the most troubled eaters: the emotionally and physically addicted eaters who need to abstain from their binge triggers and simply don't do as well if they keep torturing themselves with their addiction and constant decision-making about what to eat. If you are one of those people, I hope you can recognize how your own food preferences and decisions haven't worked for you in the past. This time, allow me to make these decisions for you. Let *me* decide what you should eat, and stick with it 100 percent. The results will be miraculous. Like thousands of others, you'll not only achieve a favorable weight, you'll feel so well and vibrantly healthy that you'll never turn back. I'll be rooting for you.

As nutritarians, it's on us to drag a resistant society with us, whether they like it or not. Change is always slow; we can't expect society to change radically overnight, but correct information lives on, and incorrect information very slowly fades away.

I hope you can be a leader and not one of those pulled along after you let your health deteriorate to a dangerous place. I hope you fix your health now, while the opportunity still presents itself. Set an example of excellent health. Know the scientific foundations of your food choices, but don't let food become a source of conflict in your life. Support others with love, compassion, and understanding, especially those who are on a one-way train to an unhealthy life, committing slow suicide with food. Your chance to be useful to others will be possible only if you are an example to them of radiant health and happiness and grant these individuals understanding, compassion, and love, in spite of their poor food choices. That doesn't mean you have to enable their poor decisions; it means that you understand them with compassion and continually contemplate what it means to have good-will for them and others. Then, hopefully, they will eventually take an interest in learning what you are so enthusiastic about. Your creative goodwill may create a crack for you to enter their world and facilitate their change.

Stand up for what's right. Be a role model; walk the walk, and don't hide your conviction about excellent nutrition. Trying to fit in, trying to be a people-pleaser when others are on an addictive, self-destructive course isn't good for them or for you. Every time you eat with another person—every dinner meeting, every party—is an opportunity to have a positive, encouraging influence on someone else. Your example of good eating, and sharing how enjoyable a healthful life can be, can eventually have a positive effect on others.

I wish you a long and pleasurable life. It can be yours.

Appendix: Considering Supplements

Once you start to eat healthfully, using supplements judiciously and conservatively is often a wise choice. Your diet may be the major part of the health pie, but it is not the whole pie. It's also necessary to assure that you aren't hurting yourself with the wrong nutritional supplements. Remember: Too little of something can be suboptimal, but too much can be as well. We have to be cautious and informed to do the right thing, because very few people understand these complicated issues.

Certain supplemental ingredients are controversial, and my comprehensive review of the available science reveals that many of the synthetic elements in typical multivitamins have, alarmingly, been linked to an increased risk of cancer. Proving a definitive link between a supplement and cancer takes many years to accomplish. Don't be persuaded by a five-year study looking at the potential cancer-promoting risks of folic acid and claiming that it's safe. Five years simply isn't long enough for the potential risk to arise. We must give heavier weight to studies that look at outcomes after ten to thirty years.

It's also still important to consider that even the healthiest diet may not supply you with the optimal amount of every potentially beneficial substance or nutrient. Supplementing those nutrients may be advantageous for long-term health.

Use supplements wisely and conservatively to assure that no deficiencies exist.

Just because almost all multivitamins contain some questionable and potentially cancer-promoting ingredients doesn't mean that all supplements are harmful or worthless. Certainly, not all supplemental ingredients are potentially harmful; many have significant benefits. A healthy diet might contain suboptimal levels of vitamins B_{12} and D, and for many people the levels of other critical elements may be similarly suboptimal. People aren't carbon copies of one another. Scientific literature points to the potential health problems that may arise from deficiency and insufficiency, and my decades spent examining the blood of thousands of patients have made clear that some people need supplementation of certain nutrients to maximize their health potential.

Traditional multivitamins, however, aren't the best answer. Some studies on multivitamins show benefits, and others don't; but it's not good science to look at studies on multivitamins as a whole because there are too many variables mixed together. Multivitamins are most often a combination of harmful substances and potentially helpful substances. My review of all the literature on the individual supplemental ingredients has led me to strongly advise against taking standard multivitamins that contain folic acid, beta-carotene, vitamin A (acetyl and retinyl palmitate), vitamin E, selenium, copper, and for men and postmenopausal women, iron.

Folic Acid

Stay away from folic acid, which is the synthetic form of folate, a member of the family of B vitamins. Synthetic folic acid found in supplements has a different chemical structure than natural folate, which is found abundantly in natural food, particularly green vegetables and beans. Your body processes folate and folic acid differently. Folic acid is about twice as absorbable as natural folate, and once absorbed it must be modified before it can act as folate.[1] Your body can convert only so much folic acid into folate, so too much folic acid enters the blood and tissues as unmodified folic acid.[2] Exactly what unmodified folic acid does in the human body is unclear, but there is evidence that it can disrupt normal folate metabolism and promote cancer growth. Taking synthetic folic acid has been linked to an increased risk of developing breast, prostate, and colorectal cancers.[3] For example, a ten-year study on women taking multivitamins concluded that those who took multivitamins containing folic acid increased their breast cancer risk by 20 to 30 percent.[4] A 2011 meta-analysis of six folic acid supplementation trials similarly found that the incidence of all cancers was 21 percent higher in the groups that received folic acid supplements.[5] In contrast, higher consumption of natural food folate helps to prevent breast, prostate, and colorectal cancers.[6] There is simply too much evidence to ignore. We must be cautious and avoid supplementing our diets with folic acid.

Fortunately, you don't really need to take extra folic acid, because natural folate is abundant in green vegetables, beans, and other plant foods. A nutritarian diet supplies you with enough folate for your body to function properly. Folate is essential for several chemical reactions related to DNA production, including methylation and repair mechanisms, crucial steps in the division of cells. Folate is also important for normal fetal development and support of normal immune function to fight against cancer.[7] Folate has become widely known for protecting against neural tube defects in developing babies.

The U.S. government and health authorities insist that women who may become pregnant take supplemental folic acid, rather than recommending that they eat green vegetables, which contain folate in addition to hundreds of other cancer-protective micronutrients. This pill-for-every-ill mentality may create new problems, such as an increase in childhood cancers and breast cancer. Every woman should be aware that no supplement can substitute for healthful eating. Eating folate-rich foods during pregnancy may also offer protection against cardiac birth defects, childhood respiratory illnesses, and childhood cancers.[8]

Since folate is most important very early on in pregnancy, the most important thing women can do to prevent neural tube defects and protect their unborn child from other health problems is to consistently eat plenty of greens and other folate-rich foods before becoming pregnant and during pregnancy. Folic acid is a weak substitute for the real thing.

Beta-Carotene

Beta-carotene—along with alpha-carotene, lutein, and lycopene—is one of more than six hundred carotenoids, the yellow, orange, and red pigments that have antioxidant activity and are present in fruits and vegetables. Beta-carotene is a provitamin A carotenoid, which means that it is converted to vitamin A in the body. Carotenoids contribute to proper immune function and vision and defend the body's tissues against oxidative damage. This helps to prevent chronic diseases and premature aging.[9]

Early observational studies have found that individuals with higher beta-carotene blood levels had lower risks of cancer, and interventional studies using beta-carotene and vitamin A supplements followed. However, beta-carotene supplements were unable to produce the beneficial effects of carotenoid-rich plant foods. In fact, supplementation with beta-carotene was associated with an increased risk of cancer and premature death.[10] A meta-analysis of many studies of antioxidant vitamin supplementation found that vitamin A supplements were associated with a 16 percent increased risk of death, beta-carotene a 7 percent increase, and vitamin E a 4 percent increase.[11] It is possible that beta-carotene from supplements could interfere with the absorption of other anticancer carotenoids, such as lutein and lycopene.[12]

The precise reason for the increased risk is not clear. What is clear, however, is that beta-carotene supplementation is a poor substitute for the more than six hundred carotenoids found in nature. It's possible for nutrients in isolation (in supplemental form) and at high doses to act differently in the body than when they are derived from foods and naturally balanced with other nutrients. A nutritarian diet style provides a more than adequate supply of carotenoids; therefore, supplemental beta-carotene and vitamin A simply are not needed—and they may be risky. We should not be taking supplements that increase the risk of disease. Get your beta-carotene from food, not supplements.

Vitamin A

Vitamin A (acetyl or retinyl palmitate) is likely the most dangerous supplement of all. In addition to the 16 percent increased risk of death found in a meta-analysis of vitamin A supplementation trials,[13] high doses of supplemental vitamin A may also increase calcium loss. It has also been linked to an increased incidence of hip fractures.[14] And excess vitamin A can cause liver damage and birth defects.[15]

Vitamin E

Vitamin E encompasses a number of similar fat-soluble compounds found primarily in nuts and seeds such as almonds, hazelnuts, and sunflower seeds. The multiple vitamin E fragments they contain, coupled with other healthful compounds, result in health benefits that you simply cannot obtain from a vitamin E supplement. When one fragment of vitamin E is isolated and supplemented, according to hundreds of studies, these benefits are lost. Similar to vitamin A and beta-carotene, vitamin E supplements were found to not be protective, and a small increase in the risk of death was reported in a recent meta-analysis.[16] Though hardly the most harmful of supplemental ingredients, vitamin E supplements do not give you the best benefit-to-risk ratio. Vitamin E is important, but it's best to get vitamin E from nuts and seeds.

Selenium

Selenium deficiency is definitely harmful and usually the result of a steady diet of refined foods, or malnourishment. It is also sometimes related to gastric bypass surgery. A nutritarian diet prevents selenium deficiency.

While selenium deficiency is harmful, too much selenium can be harmful too, which is why taking selenium in supplemental form is so risky. Recently, evidence has emerged that high selenium levels may be associated with diabetes, elevated cholesterol levels, prostate cancer, cardiovascular disease, and impaired immune and thyroid function. There is also a link between selenium excess and amyotrophic lateral sclerosis (ALS).[17] In light of these studies, I advise avoiding supplemental selenium. You will automatically get sufficient selenium from a healthy diet, so you won't need this ingredient in a supplement.

Copper and Iron

Copper and iron are essential minerals. Iron is crucial for oxygen transport in the blood, and both iron and copper take part in many of the body's vital chemical reactions. The human body stores excess iron and copper, and as we age these metals may build up and become toxic. Iron, in excess, also has pro-oxidant effects that may contribute to cardiovascular disease and cognitive decline in older adults.[18] Excess copper intake, especially when in conjunction with high saturated and *trans* fat intake, may also contribute to cardiovascular disease and accelerate cognitive decline in older adults.[19]

The most common sources of excess iron and copper are red meat and multivitamins. One of the negative health effects of red meat is due to its heme iron, which is too readily absorbed. Adequate, but not excessive, amounts of iron and copper are found in plant foods.

Excess iron is somewhat less of a concern for menstruating women compared with men because women lose some iron as a result of menstruation. Some women who have a heavier menstrual flow each month and who absorb iron less efficiently may require more iron than natural plant foods can supply. However, keep in mind that the health benefits of a nutritarian diet and lower body fat stores include reduced menstrual pain and menstrual bleeding over time, which would also reduce iron requirements. So the amount of iron menstruating women need can be relative to the amount of blood they lose each month, their dietary choices, and their differences in absorption of iron.

The primary issue for men and postmenopausal women is to not consume excess iron. Eating red meat can result in your getting too much iron, which can increase your risk of heart disease and dementia. The iron from supplements is not as well absorbed as the iron in meat, so a low-dose iron supplement may be helpful if an increased need exists from heavy menstrual flow. Low iron levels can cause fatigue, even when anemia is not present. Also, iron deficiency in infants and toddlers can retard brain development and intelligence, so it's important that pregnant and nursing mothers aren't deficient in iron. A blood test showing a ferritin level lower than 50ng/ml indicates a need for iron. Supplemental iron should be taken only when there is a deficiency or increased biological need, such as during pregnancy or in premenopausal women who are experiencing excessive bleeding.

Vitamin B_{12}

Vitamin B_{12} is involved in red blood cell production and keeps the nervous system working properly. Vitamin B_{12} deficiency can elevate the amino acid homocysteine, a risk factor for cardiovascular disease, and cause a number of serious health problems, including anemia, depression, confusion, fatigue, digestive issues, and nerve damage.[20] As we get older, our ability to absorb vitamin B_{12} from food begins to decline. In fact, about 20 percent of adults older than sixty have insufficient vitamin B_{12} levels, and insufficient B_{12} levels are associated with an increased risk of Alzheimer's disease.[21] In addition, vitamin B_{12} is made exclusively by microorganisms, which means that animal products are the only dependable source of it. Soil contains vitamin B_{12}–producing microorganisms, but since we wash produce before we eat it, most of us are unable to get sufficient vitamin B_{12} from plant foods alone. Therefore, vitamin B_{12} supplementation beyond what is found in a nutritarian diet is necessary.

Vitamin D

Vitamin D is produced by the skin in response to exposure to the sun's ultraviolet rays. It regulates bone density by increasing the intestinal absorption of calcium and promoting the activity of bone-building cells. Although it is most known for its role in bone health, recent evidence has shown that vitamin D has important functions relevant to many other aspects of human health.[22] Insufficient vitamin D levels are associated with several cancers, diabetes, cardiovascular disease, depression, and autoimmune diseases.[23] And a number of studies have now found correlations between low vitamin D levels and increased risk of death from all causes.[24] Higher blood levels of vitamin D, on the other hand, have been associated with reduced risk of several cancers.[25] One newly published study found that a doubling of vitamin D level resulted in a 20 to 23 percent reduced likelihood of mortality over thirteen years of follow-up.[26]

Because of our indoor jobs, our climate, and the risk of skin damage and skin cancer from overexposure to sunlight, it's very difficult to achieve optimal levels of vitamin D safely from the sun. Since the current Institute of Medicine recommendations on vitamin D intake fall below what many scientists believe to be an adequate daily dose for most people, most multivitamins do not contain enough vitamin D to constitute a healthy vitamin D level. In my experience, 2000 IU is an appropriate dose that most consistently brings most people into the favorable range for 25-hydroxy vitamin D on their blood test. My thorough review of all the science on this issue indicates a blood test range of 25 to 45 nanograms per milliliter is ideal. I have drawn thousands of vitamin D blood tests on patients over the years, and found severe deficiencies of vitamin D to be very common. I do recommend having a blood test every few years to determine your vitamin D level to assure adequacy and to make sure you are not taking too much supplemental vitamin D, which could also be harmful.

Zinc

A cofactor in hundreds of chemical reactions, zinc is an important contributor to gene expression, immune function, cell growth, and re-production. An adequate level of zinc is necessary for optimal resistance against infection, which is especially important for the elderly as immunity and disease resistance wane with aging. Although the zinc content of whole plant foods is adequate, zinc isn't as readily absorbed from plant sources compared with animal sources. This is because zinc-rich plant foods also contain substances, such as phytates,[27] that reduce zinc absorption. Suboptimal levels of zinc therefore are more likely to occur in people who eat low-calorie vegan and near-vegan diets. It is estimated that zinc requirements for people following a completely vegan diet are approximately 50 percent higher than for non-vegans.[28]

Zinc may be especially important for men, since blood zinc levels of men with prostate cancer tend to be lower than in healthy men, and long-term zinc supplementation has been associated with a decreased risk of advanced prostate cancer.[29] Supplementation with a low dose of zinc, 10 to 15 milligrams, seems wise.

Iodine

Iodine is involved in the production of thyroid hormones. Most plant foods are low in iodine, largely because of soil depletion. Studies have shown that iodine deficiency is common in vegans and vegetarians.[30]

Kelp, a sea vegetable, is a good source of iodine, but only a pinch (one-tenth teaspoon) is an appropriate dose. It could provide excessive amounts of iodine if the amounts consumed aren't carefully measured and limited. Since the primary source of iodine in the American diet is iodized salt, it may be important to supplement your iodine intake because a nutritarian diet minimizes added salt. Since both too little and too much iodine can have a negative effect on thyroid function, taking 150 micrograms a day is sufficient and protective.

Only the optimal choice of food can result in optimal health.

The right foods are still the only answer to excellent health because supplements can never supply the broad diversity and comprehensive array of immune system–supporting nutrients that we need for superior health and a long life. There is simply no substitute for eating nutrient-rich vegetation.

Supplements can add exposure to beneficial substances not found in optimal amounts in one's diet, but we always have to keep in mind that both deficiencies and excesses of individual nutrients can be problematic and many supplements, because they may contain higher amounts of individual nutrients than can be utilized by the body, can push people up to a harmful level of intake. Remember, even too much clean water can be harmful.

So though we should maintain adequate intake of DHA, B_{12}, zinc, iodine, and Vitamin D, we should also be aware that taking too much can also be harmful. I want you to aim for comprehensive nutritional adequacy, not excess. Modern nutritional science directs us to combine the optimal diet with the judicious use of supplements to adequately meet our needs. When you do this, you achieve a zone of excellence, rarely achieved by humans in prior generations or even in our world today, and you have a unique opportunity in human history to live better, healthier and longer than ever before.

Notes

The End of Dieting Pledge

1. Franz MJ, Van Wormer JJ, Crain AL, et al. Weight-loss outcomes: a systematic review and meta-analysis of weight-loss clinical trials with a minimum 1-year follow-up. *J Am Diet Assoc.* 2007;107(10):1755–1767.

2. Montani JP, Viecelli AK, Prévot A, Dulloo AG. Weight cycling during growth and beyond as a risk factor for later cardiovascular diseases: the "repeated overshoot" theory. *Int J Obes (Lond).* 2006;30(suppl 4):S58–66.

Introduction

1. Mokdad AH, Marks JS, Stroup DF, Gerberding JL. Actual causes of death in the United States, 2000. *JAMA.* 2004;291(10):1238–1245.

Chapter One: Toxic Hunger

1. Lennerz BS, Alsop DC, Holsen LM, et al. Effects of dietary glycemic index on brain regions related to reward and craving in men. *Am J Clin Nutr.* 2013; 98(3):641–647.

2. Science Daily. Compulsive eating shares addictive biochemical mechanism with cocaine, heroin abuse, study shows. http://www.sciencedaily.com/releases/2010/03/100328170243.htm. Published March 29, 2010. Accessed April 16, 2010.

3. Yona MA, Maugera SL, Pickavance LC. Relationships between dietary macronutrients and adult neurogenesis in the regulation of energy metabolism. *Brit J Nutr.* 2013;109(9):1573–1589.

4. Holt-Lunstad J, Smith TB, Layton JB. Social relationships and mortality risk: a meta-analytic review. *PLoS Med.* 2010;7(7):e1000316. doi: 10.1371/journal.pmed.1000316.

Chapter Two: Diet Myths Exposed

1. Biba E. Where is the next Carl Sagan? *Popular Science.* June 3, 2013, http://www.popsci.com/science/article/2013-05/not-just-facts.

2. Sacks FM, Bray GA, Carey VJ, et al. Comparison of weight-loss diets with different compositions of fat, protein, and carbohydrates. *N Engl J Med.* 2009;360(9):859–873. De Souza RJ, Bray GA, Carey VJ, et al. Effects of 4 weight-loss diets differing in fat, protein, and carbohydrate on fat mass, lean mass, visceral adipose tissue, and hepatic fat: results from the

POUNDS LOST trial. *Am J Clin Nutr.* 2012;95(3):614–625. Dansinger ML, Gleason JA, Griffith JL, et al. Comparison of the Atkins, Ornish, Weight Watchers, and Zone diets for weight loss and heart disease risk reduction: a randomized trial. *JAMA.* 2005;293(1):43–53.

3. Estruch R, Ros E, Salas-Salvadó J, et al. Primary prevention of cardiovascular disease with a Mediterranean diet. *N Engl J Med.* 2013;368:1279–1290.

4. Kramer CK, Zinman B, Retnakaran R. Are metabolically healthy overweight and obesity benign conditions? A systematic review and meta-analysis. *Ann Intern Med.* 2013;159(11):758–769.

5. Flegal KM, Kit BK, Orpana H, et al. Association of all-cause mortality with overweight and obesity using standard body mass index categories: a systematic review and meta-analysis. *JAMA.* 2013;309:71–82.

6. Singh PN, Fraser GE. Dietary risk factors for colon cancer in a low-risk population. *Am J Epidemiol.* 1998;148(8):761–774. Aune D, De Stefani E, Ronco A, et al. Legume intake and the risk of cancer: a multisite case-control study in Uruguay. *Cancer Causes Control.* 2009;20(9):1605–1615. Darmadi-Blackberry I, Wahlqvist ML, Kouris-Blazos A, et al. Legumes: the most important dietary predictor of survival in older people of different ethnicities. *Asia Pac J Clin Nutr.* 2004;13(2):217–220.

7. Chitnis MM, Yuen JS, Protheroe AS, et al. The type 1 insulin-like growth factor receptor pathway. *Clin Cancer Res.* 2008;14:6364–6370. Werner H, Bruchim I. The insulin-like growth factor-I receptor as an oncogene. *Arch Physiol Biochem.* 2009;115:58–71. Davies M, Gupta S, Goldspink G, et al. The insulin-like growth factor system and colorectal cancer: clinical and experimental evidence. *Int J Colorectal Dis.* 2006;21:201–208. Sandhu MS, Dunger DB, Giovannucci EL. Insulin, insulin-like growth factor-I (IGF-I), IGF binding proteins, their biologic interactions, and colorectal cancer. *J Natl Cancer Inst.* 2002;94:972–980. Rowlands MA, Gunnell D, Harris R, Vatten LJ, Holly JM, Martin RM. Circulating insulin-like growth factor peptides and prostate cancer risk: a systematic review and meta-analysis. *Int J Cancer.* 2009 May 15;124(10):2416–2429.

8. Bartke A. Minireview: role of the growth hormone/insulin-like growth factor system in mammalian aging. *Endocrinology.* 2005;146:3718–3723.

9. Grant WB. A Multicountry Ecological Study of Cancer Incidence Rates in 2008 with Respect to Various Risk-Modifying Factors. *Nutrients.* 2014; 6:163–189; doi:10.3390/nu6010163.

10. Fung TT, van Dam RM, Harkinson SE, et al. Low-carbohydrate diets and all-cause and cause-specific mortality: two cohort studies. *Ann Intern Med.* 2010;153:289–298.

11. Preis SR, Stampfer MJ, Spiegelman D, et al. Dietary protein and risk of ischemic heart disease in middle-aged men. *Am J Clin Nutr.* 2010;92:1265–1272.

12. Lagiou P, Sandin S, Lof M, et al. Low carbohydrate, high protein diet and incidence of cardiovascular disease in Swedish women: prospective cohort study. *BMJ*. 2012;344:e4026. doi: 10.1136/bmj.e4026.

13. Pan A, Sun Q, Bernstein AM, et al. Changes in red meat consumption and subsequent risk of type 2 diabetes mellitus: three cohorts of US men and women. *JAMA Intern Med*. 2013;173(14):1328–1335.

14. Vergnaud AC, Norat T, Romaguera D, et al. Meat consumption and prospective weight change in participants of the EPIC-PANACEA study. *Am J Clin Nutr*. 2010;92(2):398–407.

15. Fraser GE, Shavlik DJ. Ten years of life: is it a matter of choice? *Arch Intern Med*. 2001;161:1645–1652.

16. Guasch-Ferré M, Bulló M, Martínez-González MA, et al. Frequency of nut consumption and mortality risk in the PREDIMED nutrition intervention trial. *BMC Med*. 2013;11:164. doi:10.1186/1741-7015-11-164. Rohrmann S, Faeh D. Should we go nuts about nuts? *BMC Med*. 2013;11:165. doi:10.1186/1741-7015-11-165.

17. Sofi F, Vecchio S, Giuliani G, et al. Dietary habits, lifestyle and cardiovascular risk factors in a clinically healthy Italian population: the 'Florence' diet is not Mediterranean. *Eur J Clin Nutr.*. 2005;59, 584–591.

18. Romieu I, Lazcano-Ponce E, Sanchez-Zamorano LM, et al. Carbohydrates and the risk of breast cancer among Mexican women. *Cancer Epidemiol Biomarkers Prev*. 2004;13:1283–1289.

19. Salas-Salvadó J, Casas-Agustench P, Murphy MM, et al. The effect of nuts on inflammation. *Asia Pac J Clin Nutr*. 2008;17(suppl 1):333–336. Casas-Agustench P, Bulló M, Salas-Salvadó J. Nuts, inflammation and insulin resistance. *Asia Pac J Clin Nutr*. 2010;19(1):124–130. Gopinath B, Buyken AE, Flood VM, et al. Consumption of polyunsaturated fatty acids, fish, and nuts and risk of inflammatory disease mortality. *Am J Clin Nutr*. 2011;93(5):1073–1079. Ros E. Nuts and novel biomarkers of cardiovascular disease. *Am J Clin Nutr*. 2009;89(5):1649S–1656S. Kris-Etherton PM, Hu FB, Ros E, Sabaté J. The role of tree nuts and peanuts in the prevention of coronary heart disease: multiple potential mechanisms. *J Nutr*. 2008;138(9):1746S–1751S. O'Neil CE, Keast DR, Nicklas TA, Fulgoni VL III. Nut consumption is associated with decreased health risk factors for cardiovascular disease and metabolic syndrome in U.S. adults: NHANES 1999–2004. *J Am Coll Nutr*. 2011;30(6):502–510. Falasca M, Casari I. Cancer chemoprevention by nuts: evidence and promises. *Front Biosci (Schol Ed)*. 2012;1(4):109–120. González CA, Salas-Salvadó J. The potential of nuts in the prevention of cancer. *Br J Nutr*. 2006;96(suppl 2):S87–94.

20. Sala-Vila A, Romero-Mamani ES, Gilabert R, et al. Mediterranean diet and 2.4-year changes in ultrasound-assessed carotid intima-media thickness and plaque: a sub-study of the PREDIMED trial. Presented at the 81st EAS Congress, June 2–5, 2013, Lyons, France.

21. Guasch-Ferré M, Bulló M, Martínez-González MA, et al. Frequency of nut consumption and mortality risk in the PREDIMED nutrition intervention trial. *BMC Med.* 2013;11:164.

22. Rubio-Tapia A, Ludvigsson JF, Brantner TL, et al. The prevalence of celiac disease in the United States. *Am J Gastroenterol.* 2012;107(10):1538–1544.

23. Sapone A, Bai JC, Ciacci C, et al. Spectrum of gluten-related disorders: consensus on new nomenclature and classification. *BMC Med.* 2012;10:13. National Foundation for Celiac Awareness: Celiac Disease & Non-Celiac Gluten Sensitivity. http://www.celiaccentral.org/SiteData/docs/NFCA Celiac/a5c2249c6b6762ab/NFCA_CeliacDisease_vs_NonCeliacGluten Sensitivity.pdf.

24. Ornish D, Brown SE, Scherwitz LW, et al. Can lifestyle changes reverse coronary heart disease? The Lifestyle Heart Trial. *Lancet.* 1990;336(8708):129–133.

25. Esselstyn CB Jr. Updating a 12-year experience with arrest and reversal therapy for coronary heart disease (an overdue requiem for palliative cardiology). *Am J Cardiol.* 1999;84:339–341, A338.

26. Jaceldo-Siegl K, Oda K, St John C, et al. Nut intake and risk of metabolic syndrome. *FASEB J.* 2013;27:120.8. Kendall CWC, Augustin LSA, Bashyam B, et al. Effect of nuts on coronary heart disease risk factors in type 2 diabetes. *FASEB J.* 2013;27:368.5. O'Neil CE, Nicklas TA, Fulgoni VL. Tree nut consumption is associated with better diet quality, nutrient intake of select nutrients, and better measures of some cardiovascular risk factors (CVRF): National Health and Nutrition Examination Survey (NHANES) 2005–2010. *FASEB J.* 2013;27:847.13.

27. Baer HJ, Glynn RJ, Hu FB, et al. Risk factors for mortality in the nurses' health study: a competing risks analysis. *Am J Epidemiol.* 2011;173(3):319–329.

28. Fraser GE, Shavlik DJ. Ten years of life: is it a matter of choice? *Arch Intern Med.* 2001;161:1645–1652.

29. Schaefer EJ, Bongard V, Beiser AS, et al. Plasma phosphatidylcholine docosahexaenoic acid content and risk of dementia in Alzheimer disease. *Arch Neurol.* 2006;63:1545–1550.

30. Van Gelder BM, Tijhuis M, Kalmijn S, Kromhout D. Fish consumption, n-3 fatty acids, and subsequent 5-y cognitive decline in elderly men: the Zutphen Elderly Study. *Am J Clin Nutr.* 2007;85:1142–1147. Beydoun MA, Kaufman JS, Satia JA, et al. Plasma n-3 fatty acids and the risk of cognitive decline in older adults: the Atherosclerosis Risk in Communities Study. *Am J Clin Nutr.* 2007;85:1103–1011.

31. Söderberg M, Edlund C, Kristensson K, Dallner G. Fatty acid composition of brain phospholipids in aging and in Alzheimer's disease. *Lipids.* 1991;26:421–425.

32. Huang TL. Omega-3 fatty acids, cognitive decline, and Alzheimer's disease: a critical review and evaluation of the literature. *J Alzheimers Dis.* 2010;21:673–690.

33. Yurko-Mauro K, McCarthy D, Rom D, et al. Beneficial effects of docosahexaenoic acid on cognition in age-related cognitive decline. *Alzheimers Dement.* 2010;6:456–464.

34. Stonehouse W, Conlon CA, Podd J, et al. DHA supplementation improved both memory and reaction time in healthy young adults: a randomized controlled trial. *Am J Clin Nutr.* 2013;97(5):1134–1143.

35. Lewis MD, Hibbeln JR, Johnson JE, et al. Suicide deaths of active-duty US military and omega-3 fatty-acid status: a case-control comparison. *J Clin Psychiatry.* 2011;72(12):1585–1590.

36. Sublette ME, Ellis SP, Geant AL, Mann JJ. Meta-analysis of the effects of eicosapentaenoic acid in clinical trials in depression. *J Clin Psychiatry.* 2011;72(12):1577–1584.

37. Sarter B, Kelsey K, Harris W. Blood docosahexaenoic acid and eicosapentaenoic acid in vegans: associations with age and gender and effects of supplementation. Personal communication, publication pending.

38. Geppert J, Kraft V, Demmelmair H, Koletzko B. Docosahexaenoic acid supplementation in vegetarians effectively increases omega-3 index: a randomized trial. *Lipids.* 2005;40(8):807–814.

39. Hu FB, Stampfer MJ. Nut consumption and risk of coronary heart disease: a review of epidemiologic evidence. *Curr Atheroscler Rep.* 1999;1(3):204–209.

Chapter Three: The End of Dieting

1. Lauer JB, Reed GW, Hill JO. Effects of weight cycling induced by diet cycling in rats differing in susceptibility to dietary obesity. *Obes Res.* 1999;7: 215–222. Reed GW, Cox G, Yakubu F, Ding L, Hill JO. Effects of weight cycling in rats allowed a choice of diet. *Am J Physiol.* 1993;264:R35–R40.

2. Wallner SJ, Luschnigg N, Schnedl WJ, et al. Body fat distribution of overweight females with a history of weight cycling. *Int J Obes Relat Metab Disord.* 2004;28:1143–1148. Van der Kooy K, Leenen R, Seidell JC, et al. Effect of a weight cycle on visceral fat accumulation. *Am J Clin Nutr.* 1993;58:853–857.

3. Olson MB, Kelsey SF, Bittner V, et al. Weight cycling and high-density lipoprotein cholesterol in women: evidence of an adverse effect: a report from the NHLBI-sponsored WISE study. Women's Ischemia Syndrome Evaluation Study Group. *J Am Coll Cardiol.* 2000;36:1565–1571. Rubins HB, Robins SJ, Collins D, et al. Gemfibrozil for the secondary prevention of coronary heart disease in men with low levels of high-density lipoprotein cholesterol. Veterans Affairs High-Density Lipoprotein Cholesterol

Intervention Trial Study Group. *N Engl J Med.* 1999;341:410–418. Kajioka T, Tsuzuku S, Shimokata H, Sato Y. Effects of intentional weight cycling on non-obese young women. *Metabolism.* 2002;51:149–154. Antic V, Tempini A, Montani JP. Serial changes in cardiovascular and renal function of rabbits ingesting a high-fat, high-calorie diet. *Am J Hypertens.* 1999;12: 826–829. Schulz M, Liese AD, Boeing H, et al. Associations of short-term weight changes and weight cycling with incidence of essential hypertension in the EPIC-Potsdam Study. *J Hum Hypertens.* 2005;19:61–67.

4. Montani JP, Antic V, Yang Z, Dulloo A. Pathways from obesity to hypertension: from the perspective of a vicious triangle. *Int J Obes Relat Metab Disord.* 2002;26(suppl 2):S28–S38.

5. Lagiou P, Sandin S, Lof M, et al. Low carbohydrate, high protein diet and incidence of cardiovascular diseases in Swedish women: prospective cohort study. *BMJ.* 2012;344:e4026. Lagiou P, Sandin S, Weiderpass E, et al. Low carbohydrate, high protein diet and mortality in a cohort of Swedish women. *J Intern Med.* 2007;261:366–374.

6. Lagiou P, Sandin S, Lof M, et al. Low carbohydrate-high protein diet and incidence of cardiovascular diseases in Swedish women: prospective cohort study. *BMJ.* 2012;344:e4026. Lagiou P, Sandin S, Weiderpass E, et al. Low carbohydrate-high protein diet and mortality in a cohort of Swedish women. *J Intern Med.* 2007;261:366–374.

7. Isner JM, Sours HE, Paris AL, et al. Sudden, unexpected death in avid dieters using the liquid-protein-modified-fast diet. Observations in 17 patients and the role of the prolonged QT interval. *Circulation.* 1979;60(6):1401–1412.

8. Stevens A, Robinson P, Turpin J, et al. Sudden Cardiac Death of an Adolescent During [Atkins] Dieting. *Southern Medical Journal.* 95(2002):1047.

9. Tseng M, Olufade TO, Evers KA, Byrne C. Adolescent lifestyle factors and adult breast density in US Chinese immigrant women. *Nutr Cancer.* 2011; 63(3):342–349. Berkey CS, Frazier AL, Gardner JD, Colditz GA. Adolescence and breast carcinoma risk. *Cancer.* 1999;85(11):2400–2409.

10. Cui X, Dai Q, Tseng M, et al. Dietary Patterns and Breast Cancer Risk in the Shanghai Breast Cancer Study. *Cancer Epidemiol Biomarkers Prev.* 2007;16:1443–1448.

11. Reis JP, Loria CM, Lewis CE, et al. Association between duration of overall and abdominal obesity beginning in young adulthood and coronary artery calcification in middle age. *JAMA.* 2013;310(3):280–288.

12. Calle EE, Kaaks R. Overweight, obesity and cancer: epidemiological evidence and proposed mechanisms. *Nat Rev Cancer.* 2004;4:579–591.

13. Rastmanesh R. High polyphenol, low probiotic diet for weight loss because of intestinal microbiota interaction. *Chem Biol Interact.* 2011;189(1-2):1–8.

14. Jeffery IB, O'Toole PW. Diet-microbiota interactions and their implications for healthy living. *Nutrients*. 2013;5(1):234–252. Koeth RA, Wang Z, Levison BS, et al. Intestinal microbiota metabolism of l-carnitine, a nutrient in red meat, promotes atherosclerosis. *Nat Med*. 2013;19(5):576–585.

15. Andersen C, Rayalam S, Della-Fera MA, Baile CA. Phytochemicals and adipogenesis. *Biofactors*. 2010;36(6):415–422. Kim HK, Kim JN, Han SN, et al. Black soybean anthocyanins inhibit adipocyte differentiation in 3T3-L1 cells. *Nutr Res*. 2012;32(10):770–777. Rayalam S, Della-Fera MA, Baile CA. Phytochemicals and regulation of the adipocyte life cycle. *J Nutr Biochem*. 2008;19(11):717–726. Baile CA, Yang JY, Rayalam S, et al. Effect of resveratrol on fat mobilization. *Ann NY Acad Sci*. 2011;1215:40–47. Rayalam S, Della-Fera MA, Yang JY, et al. Resveratrol potentiates genistein's antiadipogenic and proapoptotic effects in 3T3-L1 adipocytes. *J Nutr*. 2007;137(12):2668–2673.

Chapter Four: The Power of Real Food

1. Moore SC, Carter LM, van Goozen S. Confectionery consumption in childhood and adult violence. *Br J Psychiatry*. 2009;195(4):366–367. Gesch CB. Influence of supplementary vitamins, minerals and essential fatty acids on the antisocial behaviour of young adult prisoners: Randomised, placebo-controlled trial. *Brit J Psych*. 2002 2002/07/01;181(1): 22–28. Virkkunen M, Huttunen MO. Evidence for abnormal glucose tolerance test among violent offenders. *Neuropsychobiology*. 1982;8(1):30–34. PubMed PMID: 7057987. Golomb BA, Evans MA, White HL, et al. Trans fat consumption and aggression. *PloS one*. 2012;7(3):e32175. PubMed PMID: 22403632. Pubmed Central PMCID: 3293881. Yau PL, Castro MG, Tagani A, et al. Obesity and metabolic syndrome and functional and structural brain impairments in adolescence. *Pediatrics*. 20102;130:e856–864. Thaler JP, Yi C-X, Schur EA, et al. Obesity is associated with hypothalamic injury in rodents and humans. *J Clin Invest*. 2012 2012/01/03;122(1): 153–162. Northstone K, Joinson C, Emmett P, et al. Are dietary patterns in childhood associated with IQ at 8 years of age? A population-based cohort study. *J Epidemiol Community Health*. 2012 Jul;66(7):624–628. PubMed PMID: 21300993.

2. Science Daily. Consumers over age 50 should consider cutting copper and iron intake, report suggests. http://www.sciencedaily.com/releases/2010/01 /100120113553.htm. Published January 22, 2010; accessed January 29, 2010. Brewer GJ. Risks of copper and iron toxicity during aging in humans. *Chem Res Toxicol*. 2010;23(2):319–326. Brewer GJ. Iron and copper toxicity in diseases of aging, particularly atherosclerosis and Alzheimer's disease. *Exp Biol Med*. 2007;232(2):323–335. Kidd PM. Neurodegeneration from mitochondrial insufficiency: Nutrients, stem cells, growth factors, and prospects for brain rebuilding using integrative management. *Altern Med Rev*. 2005;10(4):268–293. Morris MC, Evans DA, Tangney CC, et al. Dietary copper and high saturated and trans fat intakes associated with cognitive decline. *Arch Neurol*. 2006;63(8):1085–1088.

3. Milton K. Back to basics: why foods of wild primates have relevance for modern human health. *Nutrition.* 2000;16(7/8):480–484.

4. Richer SP. Randomized, double-blind, placebo-controlled study of zeaxanthin and visual function in patients with atrophic age-related macular degeneration. *Optometry.* 2011;82(11);667–680. Semba RD. Are lutein and zeaxanthin conditionally essential nutrients for eye health? *Med Hypotheses.* 2003;61(4):465–472. Willett W, Sampson L, Stampfer M, et al. Reproducibility and validity of a semiquantitative food frequency questionnaire. *Am J Epidemiol.* 1985;122:51–65. Delcourt C, Carrière I, Delage M, et al. Plasma lutein and zeaxanthin and other carotenoids as modifiable risk factors for age-related maculopathy and cataract: the POLA Study. *Invest Ophthalmol Vis Sci.* 2006;47:2329–2335.

5. Higdon J, Delage B, Williams D, et al. Cruciferous vegetables and human cancer risk: epidemiologic evidence and mechanistic basis. *Pharmacol Res.* 2007;55:224–236.

6. Cornblatt BS, Ye L, Dinkova-Kostova AT, et al. Preclinical and clinical evaluation of sulforaphane for chemoprevention in the breast. *Carcinogenesis.* 2007;28:1485–1490.

7. Zhang CX, Ho SC, Chen YM, et al. Greater vegetable and fruit intake is associated with a lower risk of breast cancer among Chinese women. *Int J Cancer.* 2009;125:181–188.

8. Bosetti C, Filomeno M, Riso P, et al. Cruciferous vegetables and cancer risk in a network of case-control studies. *Ann Oncol.* 2012;23(8):2198–2203.

9. Nechuta SJ, Lu W, Cai H, et al. Cruciferous vegetable intake after diagnosis of breast cancer and survival: a report from the Shanghai Breast Cancer Survival study. Presented at the Annual Meeting of the American Association for Cancer Research; March 31–April 4, 2012; Chicago. Abstract no. LB-322.

10. Thomson CA, Rock CL, Thompson PA, et al. Vegetable intake is associated with reduced breast cancer recurrence in tamoxifen users: a secondary analysis from the Women's Healthy Eating and Living Study. *Breast Cancer Res Treat.* 2011;125:519–527.

11. Garg M, Garg C, Mukherjee PK, Suresh B. Antioxidant potential of Lactuca sativa. *Anc Sci Life.* 2004;24(1):6–10. Mulabagal V, Ngouajio M, Nair A, et al. In vitro evaluation of red and green lettuce (Lactuca sativa) for functional food properties. *Food Chem.* 2010;118(2):300–306. Serafini M, Bugianesi R, Salucci M, et al. Effect of acute ingestion of fresh and stored lettuce (Lactuca sativa) on plasma total antioxidant capacity and antioxidant levels in human subjects. *Br J Nutr.* 2002;88(6):615–623. Gridling M, Popescu R, Kopp B, et al. Anti-leukaemic effects of two extract types of Lactuca sativa correlate with the activation of Chk2, induction of p21, downregulation of cyclin D1 and acetylation of alpha-tubulin. *Oncol Rep.* 2010;23(4):1145–1151.

12. Zhao J, Moore AN, Redell JB, et al. Enhancing expression of Nrf2-driven genes protects the blood brain barrier after brain injury. *J Neurosci.* 2007;27:10240–10248. Carter P, Gray LJ, Troughton J, et al. Fruit and vegetable intake and incidence of type 2 diabetes mellitus: systematic review and meta-analysis. *BMJ.* 2010;341:c4229. Lundberg JO, Carlstrom M, Larsen FJ, et al. Roles of dietary inorganic nitrate in cardiovascular health and disease. *Cardiovasc Res.* 2011;89:525–532. Higdon J, Delage B, Williams D, et al. Cruciferous vegetables and human cancer risk: epidemiologic evidence and mechanistic basis. *Pharmacol Res.* 2007;55:224–236. Stringham JM, Bovier ER, Wong JC, et al. The influence of dietary lutein and zeaxanthin on visual performance. *J Food Sci.* 2010;75:R24–R29.

13. Mulabagal V, Ngouajio M, Nair A, et al. In vitro evaluation of red and green lettuce (Lactuca sativa) for functional food properties. *Food Chem.* 2010;118(2):300–306.

14. World Cancer Research Fund, American Institute for Cancer Research. Expert report. Food, nutrition, physical activity, and the prevention of cancer: a global perspective. World Cancer Research Fund; 2007.

15. Bessaoud F, Daurès JP, Gerber M. Dietary factors and breast cancer risk: a case control study among a population in Southern France. *Nutr Cancer.* 2008;60(2):177–187. Link LB, Potter JD. Raw versus cooked vegetables and cancer risk. *Cancer Epidemiol Biomarkers Prev.* 2004;13(9):1422–1435.

16. Cox BD, Whichelow MJ, Prevost AT. Seasonal consumption of salad vegetables and fresh fruit in relation to the development of cardiovascular disease and cancer. *Public Health Nutr.* 2000;3(1):19–29. Lockheart MS, Steffen LM, Rebnord HM, et al. Dietary patterns, food groups and myocardial infarction: a case-control study. *Brit J Nutr.* 2007;98(2):380–387. Oude Griep LM, Verschuren WM, Kromhout D, et al. Raw and processed fruit and vegetable consumption and 10-year stroke incidence in a population-based cohort study in the Netherlands. *Eur J Clin Nutr.* 2011;65(7):791–799.

17. Rolls BJ, Roe LS, Meengs JS. Salad and satiety: energy density and portion size of a first-course salad affect energy intake at lunch. *J Am Diet Assoc.* 2004;104(10):1570–1576. Roe LS, Meengs JS, Rolls BJ. Salad and satiety: the effect of timing of salad consumption on meal energy intake. *Appetite.* 2012;58(1):242–248.

18. Behall KM, Howe JC. Effect of long-term consumption of amylose vs amylopectin starch on metabolic variables in human subjects. *Am J Clin Nutr.* 1995;61:334–340. Marlett JA, McBurney MI, Slavin JL. Position of the American Dietetic Association: health implications of dietary fiber. *J Am Diet Assoc.* 2002;102:993–1000. Aller EE, Abete I, Astrup A, et al. Starches, sugars and obesity. *Nutrients.* 2011;3:341–369. Wylie-Rosett J, Segal-Isaacson CJ, Segal-Isaacson A. Carbohydrates and increases in obesity: does the type of carbohydrate make a difference? *Obes Res.* 2004;12(suppl 2):124S–129S.

19. Bednar GE, Patil AR, Murray SM, et al. Starch and fiber fractions in selected food and feed ingredients affect their small intestinal digestibility and

fermentability and their large bowel fermentability in vitro in a canine model. *J Nutr*. 2001;131:276–286. Muir JG, O'Dea K. Measurement of resistant starch: factors affecting the amount of starch escaping digestion in vitro. *Am J Clin Nutr*. 1992;56:123–127.

20. Jenkins DJ, Kendall CW, Augustin LS, et al. Effect of legumes as part of a low glycemic index diet on glycemic control and cardiovascular risk factors in type 2 diabetes mellitus: a randomized controlled trial. *Arch Intern Med*. 2012;172(21):1653–1660.

21. Halton TL, Willett WC, Liu S, et al. Potato and french fry consumption and risk of type 2 diabetes in women. *Am J Clin Nutr*. 2006;83:284–290.

22. Streppel MT, Arends LR, van't Veer P, et al. Dietary fiber and blood pressure: a meta-analysis of randomized placebo-controlled trials. *Arch Intern Med*. 2005;165:150–156. Houston MC. The importance of potassium in managing hypertension. *Curr Hypertens Rep*. 2011;13:309–317. Houston M. The role of magnesium in hypertension and cardiovascular disease. *J Clin Hypertens*. 2011;13:843–847. DeFronzo RA, Cooke CR, Andres R, et al. The effect of insulin on renal handling of sodium, potassium, calcium, and phosphate in man. *J Clin Invest*. 1975;55:845–855. Chiasson JL, Josse RG, Gomis R, et al. Acarbose treatment and the risk of cardiovascular disease and hypertension in patients with impaired glucose tolerance: the STOP-NIDDM trial. *JAMA*. 2003;290:486–494.

23. Papanikolaou Y, Fulgoni VL. Bean consumption is associated with greater nutrient intake, reduced systolic blood pressure, lower body weight, and a smaller waist circumference in adults: results from the National Health and Nutrition Examination Survey 1999–2002. *J Am Coll Nutr*. 2008;27:569–576. Bazzano LA, Thompson AM, Tees MT, et al. Non-soy legume consumption lowers cholesterol levels: a meta-analysis of randomized controlled trials. *Nutr Metab Cardiovasc Dis*. 2011;21:94–103.

24. Hamer HM, Jonkers D, Venema K, et al. Review article: the role of butyrate on colonic function. *Aliment Pharmacol Ther*. 2008;27:104–119. O'Keefe SJ, Ou J, Aufreiter S, et al. Products of the colonic microbiota mediate the effects of diet on colon cancer risk. *J Nutr*. 2009;139:2044–2048. Singh PN, Fraser GE. Dietary risk factors for colon cancer in a low-risk population. *Am J Epidemiol*. 1998;148:761–774.

25. Aune D, De Stefani E, Ronco A, et al. Legume intake and the risk of cancer: a multisite case-control study in Uruguay. *Cancer Causes Control*. 2009;20:1605–1615. Bao PP, Shu XO, Zheng Y, et al. Fruit, vegetable, and animal food intake and breast cancer risk by hormone receptor status. *Nutr Cancer*. 2012;64:806–819.

26. Dong JY, He K, Wang P, Qin LQ. Dietary fiber intake and risk of breast cancer: a meta-analysis of prospective cohort studies. *Am J Clin Nutr*. 2011;94(3):900–905.

27. Powolny A, Singh S. Multitargeted prevention and therapy of cancer by diallyl trisulfide and related Allium vegetable-derived organosulfur compounds. *Cancer Lett.* 2008;269:305–314. Ginter E, Simko V. Garlic (Allium sativum L.) and cardiovascular diseases. *Bratisl Lek Listy.* 2010;111:452–456. Taj Eldin IM, Ahmed EM, Elwahab HMA. Preliminary study of the clinical hypoglycemic effects of *Allium cepa* (red onion) in type 1 and type 2 diabetic patients. *Environ Health Insights.* 2010;4:71–77.

28. Slimestad R, Fossen T, Vagen IM. Onions: a source of unique dietary flavonoids. *J Agric Food Chem.* 2007;55:10067–10080. Miyamoto S, Yasui Y, Ohigashi H, et al. Dietary flavonoids suppress azoxymethane-induced colonic preneoplastic lesions in male C57BL/KsJ-db/db mice. *Chem Biol Interact.* 2010;183:276–283. Shan BE, Wang MX, Li RQ. Quercetin inhibits human SW480 colon cancer growth in association with inhibition of cyclin D1 and surviving expression through Wnt/beta-catenin signaling pathway. *Cancer Invest.* 2009;27:604–612.

29. Galeone C, Pelucchi C, Levi F, et al. Onion and garlic use and human cancer. *Am J Clin Nutr.* 2006;84:1027–1032.

30. Modem S, Dicarlo SE, Reddy TR. Fresh garlic extract induces growth arrest and morphological differentiation of MCF7 breast cancer cells. *Genes Cancer.* 2012;3:177–186. Na HK, Kim EH, Choi MA, et al. Diallyl trisulfide induces apoptosis in human breast cancer cells through ROS-mediated activation of JNK and AP-1. *Biochem Pharmacol.* 2012;84(10):1241–1250. Malki A, El-Saadani M, Sultan AS. Garlic constituent diallyl trisulfide induced apoptosis in MCF7 human breast cancer cells. *Cancer Biol Ther.* 2009;8:2175–2185.

31. Ravasco P, Aranha MM, Borralho PM, et al. Colorectal cancer: can nutrients modulate NF-kappaB and apoptosis? *Clin Nutr.* 2010;29:42–46. Pierini R, Gee JM, Belshaw NJ, et al. Flavonoids and intestinal cancers. *Brit J Nutr.* 2008;99(suppl 1):ES53–59.

32. Yu L, Fernig DG, Smith JA, et al. Reversible inhibition of proliferation of epithelial cell lines by *Agaricus bisporus* (edible mushroom) lectin. *Cancer Res* 1993;53:4627–4632.

33. Borchers AT, Krishnamurthy A, Keen CL, et al. The immunobiology of mushrooms. *Exp Biol Med.* 2008;233:259–276.

34. Zhang M, Huang J, Xie X, et al. Dietary intakes of mushrooms and green tea combine to reduce the risk of breast cancer in Chinese women. *Int J Cancer.* 2009;124:1404–1408.

35. Hong SA, Kim K, Nam SJ, et al. A case-control study on the dietary intake of mushrooms and breast cancer risk among Korean women. *Int J Cancer.* 2008;122:919–923. Shin A, Kim J, Lim SY, et al. Dietary mushroom intake and the risk of breast cancer based on hormone receptor status. *Nutr Cancer.* 2010;62:476–483.

36. Cao QZ, Lin ZB. Antitumor and anti-angiogenic activity of Ganoderma lucidum polysaccharides peptide. *Acta Pharmacol Sin.* 2004;25:833–838. Lee JS, Park BC, Ko YJ, et al. Grifola frondosa (maitake mushroom) water extract inhibits vascular endothelial growth factor-induced angiogenesis through inhibition of reactive oxygen species and extracellular signal-regulated kinase phosphorylation. *J Med Food.* 2008;11:643–651. Chang HH, Hsieh KY, Yeh CH, et al. Oral administration of an Enoki mushroom protein FVE activates innate and adaptive immunity and induces anti-tumor activity against murine hepatocellular carcinoma. *Int Immunopharmacol.* 2010;10:239–246.

37. Hara M, Hanaoka T, Kobayashi M, et al. Cruciferous vegetables, mushrooms, and gastrointestinal cancer risks in a multicenter, hospital-based case-control study in Japan. *Nutr Cancer.* 2003;46:138–147. Zhang CX, Ho SC, Chen YM, et al. Greater vegetable and fruit intake is associated with a lower risk of breast cancer among Chinese women. *Int J Cancer.* 2009;125:181–188. Martin KR, Brophy SK. Commonly consumed and specialty dietary mushrooms reduce cellular proliferation in MCF-7 human breast cancer cells. *Exp Biol Med.* 2010;235:1306–1314. Fang N, Li Q, Yu S, et al. Inhibition of growth and induction of apoptosis in human cancer cell lines by an ethyl acetate fraction from shiitake mushrooms. *J Altern Complement Med.* 2006;12:125–132. Ng ML, Yap AT. Inhibition of human colon carcinoma development by lentinan from shiitake mushrooms (Lentinus edodes). *J Altern Complement Med.* 2002;8:581–589. Adams LS, Phung S, Wu X, et al. White button mushroom (Agaricus bisporus) exhibits antiproliferative and proapoptotic properties and inhibits prostate tumor growth in athymic mice. *Nutr Cancer.* 2008;60:744–756. Lakshmi B, Ajith TA, Sheena N, et al. Antiperoxidative, anti-inflammatory, and antimutagenic activities of ethanol extract of the mycelium of Ganoderma lucidum occurring in South India. *Teratog Carcinog Mutagen.* 2003;suppl 1:85–97. Lin ZB, Zhang HN. Anti-tumor and immuno-regulatory activities of Ganoderma lucidum and its possible mechanisms. *Acta Pharmacol Sin.* 2004;25:1387–1395.

38. Poddar KH, Ames M, Chen H, et al. Positive effect of white button mushrooms when substituted for meat on body weight and composition changes during weight loss and weight maintenance: a one-year randomized clinical trial. *FASEB J.* 2013;27:852.4.

39. Su CH, Lai MN, Ng LT. Inhibitory effects of medicinal mushrooms on α-amylase and α-glucosidase—enzymes related to hyperglycemia. *Food Funct.* 2013;4(4):644–649.

40. Varshney J, Ooi JH, Jayarao BM, et al. White button mushrooms increase microbial diversity and accelerate the resolution of Citrobacter rodentium infection in mice. *J Nutr.* 2013;143(4):526–532.

41. Jeong SC, Koyyalamudi SR, Pang G. Dietary intake of Agaricus bisporus white button mushroom accelerates salivary immunoglobulin A secretion in healthy volunteers. *Nutrition.* 2012;28(5):527–531.

42. Toth B, Erickson J. Cancer induction in mice by feeding of the uncooked cultivated mushroom of commerce Agaricus bisporus. *Cancer Res.* 1986; 46:4007–4011. Schulzová V, Hajslová J, Peroutka R, et al. Influence of storage and household processing on the agaritine content of the cultivated Agaricus mushroom. *Food Addit Contam.* 2002;19:853–862.

43. Huxley RR, Neil HA. The relation between dietary flavonol intake and coronary heart disease mortality: a meta-analysis of prospective cohort studies. *Eur J Clin Nutr.* 2003;57:904–908. Knekt P, Kumpulainen J, Jarvinen R, et al. Flavonoid intake and risk of chronic diseases. *Am J Clin Nutr.* 2002;76:560–568. Mursu J, Voutilainen S, Nurmi T, et al. Flavonoid intake and the risk of ischaemic stroke and CVD mortality in middle-aged Finnish men: the Kuopio Ischaemic Heart Disease Risk Factor Study. *Brit J Nutr.* 2008;100:890–895. Mink PJ, Scrafford CG, Barraj LM, et al. Flavonoid intake and cardiovascular disease mortality: a prospective study in postmenopausal women. *Am J Clin Nutr.* 2007;85:895–909.

44. Bazzano LA, Li TY, Joshipura KJ, et al. Intake of fruit, vegetables, and fruit juices and risk of diabetes in women. *Diabetes Care.* 2008;31:1311–1317. Hannum SM. Potential impact of strawberries on human health: a review of the science. *Crit Rev Food Sci Nutr.* 2004;44:1–17. Joseph JA, Shukitt-Hale B, Willis LM. Grape juice, berries, and walnuts affect brain aging and behavior. *J Nutr.* 2009;139:1813S–1817S. Cassidy A, O'Reilly EJ, Kay C, et al. Habitual intake of flavonoid subclasses and incident hypertension in adults. *Am J Clin Nutr.* 2011;93:338–347. Devore EE, Kang JH, Breteler MM, et al. Dietary intakes of berries and flavonoids in relation to cognitive decline. *Ann Neurol.* 2012;72(1):135–143.

45. Smart RC, Huang MT, Chang RL, et al. Disposition of the naturally occurring antimutagenic plant phenol, ellagic acid, and its synthetic derivatives, 3-O-decylellagic acid and 3,3'-di-O-methylellagic acid in mice. *Carcinogenesis.* 1986;7:1663–1667. Smart RC, Huang MT, Chang RL, et al. Effect of ellagic acid and 3-O-decylellagic acid on the formation of benzo[a]pyrene-derived DNA adducts in vivo and on the tumorigenicity of 3-methylcholanthrene in mice. *Carcinogenesis.* 1986;7:1669–1675.

46. Stoner GD, Wang LS, Casto BC. Laboratory and clinical studies of cancer chemoprevention by antioxidants in berries. *Carcinogenesis.* 2008; 29:1665–1674.

47. Kim ND, Mehta R, Yu W, et al. Chemopreventive and adjuvant therapeutic potential of pomegranate (Punica granatum) for human breast cancer. *Breast Cancer Res Treat.* 2002;71:203–217. Kohno H, Suzuki R, Yasui Y, et al. Pomegranate seed oil rich in conjugated linolenic acid suppresses chemically induced colon carcinogenesis in rats. *Cancer Sci.* 2004;95:481–486. Kawaii S, Lansky EP. Differentiation-promoting activity of pomegranate (Punica granatum) fruit extracts in HL-60 human promyelocytic leukemia cells. *J Med Food.* 2004;7:13–18.

48. Roy S, Khanna S, Alessio HM, et al. Anti-angiogenic property of edible berries. *Free Radic Res.* 2002;36:1023–1031. Khan N, Afaq F, Kweon MH, et al. Oral consumption of pomegranate fruit extract inhibits growth and progression of primary lung tumors in mice. *Cancer Res.* 2007;67:3475–3482. Toi M, Bando H, Ramachandran C, et al. Preliminary studies on the anti-angiogenic potential of pomegranate fractions in vitro and in vivo. *Angiogenesis.* 2003;6:121–128. Sartippour MR, Seeram NP, Rao JY, et al. Ellagitannin-rich pomegranate extract inhibits angiogenesis in prostate cancer in vitro and in vivo. *Int J Oncol.* 2008;32:475–480. Panchal SK, Ward L, Brown L. Ellagic acid attenuates high-carbohydrate, high-fat diet-induced metabolic syndrome in rats. *Eur J Nutr.* 2013;52(2):559–568. Edirisinghe I, Banaszewski K, Cappozzo J, et al. Strawberry anthocyanin and its association with postprandial inflammation and insulin. *Br J Nutr.* 2011;106:913–922. Adams LS, Seeram NP, Aggarwal BB, et al. Pomegranate juice, total pomegranate ellagitannins, and punicalagin suppress inflammatory cell signaling in colon cancer cells. *J Agric Food Chem.* 2006;54:980–985.

49. Adams LS, Zhang Y, Seeram NP, et al. Pomegranate ellagitannin-derived compounds exhibit antiproliferative and antiaromatase activity in breast cancer cells in vitro. *Cancer Prev Res.* 2010;3:108–113.

50. American Association for Cancer Research. Strawberries may slow precancerous growth in esophagus. http://aacrnews.wordpress.com/2011/04/06/strawberries-may-slow-precancerous-growth-in-esophagus/. Published April 6, 2011.

51. Boqué N, de la Iglesia R, de la Garza AL, et al. Prevention of diet-induced obesity by apple polyphenols in Wistar rats through regulation of adipocyte gene expression and DNA methylation patterns. *Mol Nutr Food Res.* 2013;57(8):1473–1478. doi: 10.1002/mnfr.201200686. Chang JJ, Hsu MJ, Huang HP, et al. Mulberry anthocyanins inhibit oleic acid induced lipid accumulation by reduction of lipogenesis and promotion of hepatic lipid clearance. *J Agric Food Chem.* 2013;61(25):6069–6076.

52. Jeffery IB, O'Toole PW. Diet-microbiota interactions and their implications for healthy living. *Nutrients.* 2013;5(1):234–52. Tuohy KM, Conterno L, Gasperotti M, Viola R. Up-regulating the human intestinal microbiome using whole plant foods, polyphenols, and/or fiber. *J Agric Food Chem.* 2012;60(36):8776–8782. Pray L, Pillsbury L, Tomayko E. The Human Microbiome, Diet, and Health: Workshop Summary Institute of Medicine (US) Food Forum. Food and Nutrition Board (FNB) Washington (DC): National Academies Press (US); 2013.

53. Cassidy A, O'Reilly EJ, Kay C, et al. Habitual intake of flavonoid subclasses and incident hypertension in adults. *Am J Clin Nutr.* 2011;93(2):338–347.

54. Cassidy A, Mukamal KJ, Liu L, et al. High anthocyanin intake is associated with a reduced risk of myocardial infarction in young and middle-aged women. *Circulation.* 2013;127:188–196.

55. Galleano M, Pechanova O, Fraga CG. Hypertension, nitric oxide, oxidants, and dietary plant polyphenols. *Curr Pharm Biotechnol.* 2010;11:837–848. Basu A, Rhone M, Lyons TJ. Berries: emerging impact on cardiovascular health. *Nutr Rev.* 2010;68:168–177. Chong MF, Macdonald R, Lovegrove JA. Fruit polyphenols and CVD risk: a review of human intervention studies. *Brit J Nutr.* 2010;104(suppl 3):S28–S39. Basu A, Du M, Leyva MJ, et al. Blueberries decrease cardiovascular risk factors in obese men and women with metabolic syndrome. *J Nutr.* 2010;140:1582–1587.

56. Devore EE, Kang JH, Breteler MM, et al. Dietary intakes of berries and flavonoids in relation to cognitive decline. *Ann Neurol.* 2012;72(1):135–143.

57. Joseph JA, Shukitt-Hale B, Willis LM. Grape juice, berries, and walnuts affect brain aging and behavior. *J Nutr.* 2009;139:1813S–1817S. Ma Y, Njike VY, Millet J, et al. Effects of walnut consumption on endothelial function in type 2 diabetic subjects: a randomized controlled crossover trial. *Diabetes Care.* 2010;33:227–232.

58. Mattes RD, Dreher ML. Nuts and healthy body weight maintenance mechanisms. *Asia Pac J Clin Nutr.* 2010;19:137–141.

59. Thompson LU, Chen JM, Li T, et al. Dietary flaxseed alters tumor biological markers in postmenopausal breast cancer. *Clin Cancer Res.* 2005; 11:3828–3835.

60. McCann SE, Thompson LU, Nie J, et al. Dietary lignan intakes in relation to survival among women with breast cancer: the Western New York Exposures and Breast Cancer (WEB) Study. *Breast Cancer Res Treat.* 2010;122(1):229–235.

61. Connor WE. Importance of n-3 fatty acids in health and disease. *Am J Clin Nutr.* 2000;71(suppl 1):171S–175S.

62. Yehuda S, Rabinovitz S, Mostofsky DI. Mixture of essential fatty acids lowers test anxiety. *Nutr Neurosci.* 2005;8(4):265–267. Lucas M, Mirzaei F, O'Reilly EJ, et al. Dietary intake of n-3 and n-6 fatty acids and the risk of clinical depression in women: a 10-y prospective follow-up study. *Am J Clin Nutr.* 2011;93(6):1337–1343.

63. Shardell MD, Alley DE, Hicks GE, et al. Low-serum carotenoid concentrations and carotenoid interactions predict mortality in US adults: the Third National Health and Nutrition Examination Survey. *Nutr Res.* 2011;31:178–189.

64. Canene-Adams K, Campbell JK, Zaripheh S, et al. The tomato as a functional food. *J Nutr.* 2005;135:1226–1230.

65. Van Breemen RB, Pajkovic N. Multitargeted therapy of cancer by lycopene. *Cancer Lett.* 2008;269:339–351.

66. Rizwan M, Rodriquez-Blanco I, Harbottle A, et al. Tomato paste rich in lycopene protects against cutaneous photodamage in humans in vivo. *Br J Dermatol.* 2011;164(1):154–162.

67. Rissanen TH, Voutilainen S, Nyyssönen K, et al. Low serum lycopene concentration is associated with an excess incidence of acute coronary events and stroke: the Kuopio Ischaemic Heart Disease Risk Factor Study. *Br J Nutr.* 2001;85:749–754. Rissanen T, Voutilainen S, Nyyssönen K, et al. Lycopene, atherosclerosis, and coronary heart disease. *Exp Biol Med.* 2002;227:900–907. Rissanen TH, Voutilainen S, Nyyssönen K, et al. Serum lycopene concentrations and carotid atherosclerosis: the Kuopio Ischaemic Heart Disease Risk Factor Study. *Am J Clin Nutr.* 2003;77:133–138.

68. Sesso HD, Buring JE, Norkus EP, et al. Plasma lycopene, other carotenoids, and retinol and the risk of cardiovascular disease in women. *Am J Clin Nutr.* 2004;79:47–53.

69. Hak AE, Ma J, Powell CB, et al. Prospective study of plasma carotenoids and tocopherols in relation to risk of ischemic stroke. *Stroke.* 2004;35:1584–1588.

70. Karppi J, Laukkanen JA, Sivenius J, et al. Serum lycopene decreases the risk of stroke in men: a population-based follow-up study. *Neurology.* 2012;79:1540–1547.

71. Karppi J, Laukkanen JA, Makikallio TH, et al. Low serum lycopene and beta-carotene increase risk of acute myocardial infarction in men. *Eur J Public Health.* 2012;22(6):835–840.

72. Silaste ML, Alfthan G, Aro A, et al. Tomato juice decreases LDL cholesterol levels and increases LDL resistance to oxidation. *Br J Nutr.* 2007;98:1251–1258. Burton-Freeman B, Talbot J, Park E, et al. Protective activity of processed tomato products on postprandial oxidation and inflammation: a clinical trial in healthy weight men and women. *Mol Nutr Food Res.* 2012;56:622–631. Hadley CW, Clinton SK, Schwartz SJ. The consumption of processed tomato products enhances plasma lycopene concentrations in association with a reduced lipoprotein sensitivity to oxidative damage. *J Nutr.* 2003;133:727–732.

73. Xaplanteris P, Vlachopoulos C, Pietri P, et al. Tomato paste supplementation improves endothelial dynamics and reduces plasma total oxidative status in healthy subjects. *Nutr Res.* 2012;32:390–394.

74. Ried K, Fakler P. Protective effect of lycopene on serum cholesterol and blood pressure: meta-analyses of intervention trials. *Maturitas.* 2011;68:299–310.

75. Palozza P, Parrone N, Catalano A, et al. Tomato lycopene and inflammatory cascade: basic interactions and clinical implications. *Curr Med Chem.* 2010;17:2547–2563. Palozza P, Parrone N, Simone RE, et al. Lycopene in atherosclerosis prevention: an integrated scheme of the potential mechanisms of action from cell culture studies. *Arch Biochem Biophys.* 2010;504:26–33.

76. USDA, Economic Research Service. Food availability (per capita) data system. http://www.ers.usda.gov/data-products/food-availability-(per -capita)-data-system.aspx.

77. Brown MJ, Ferruzzi MG, Nguyen ML, et al. Carotenoid bioavailability is higher from salads ingested with full-fat than with fat-reduced salad dressings as measured with electrochemical detection. *Am J Clin Nutr.* 2004;80:396–403.

78. Van het Hof KH, de Boer BC, Tijburg LB, et al. Carotenoid bioavailability in humans from tomatoes processed in different ways determined from the carotenoid response in the triglyceride-rich lipoprotein fraction of plasma after a single consumption and in plasma after four days of consumption. *J Nutr.* 2000;130:1189–1196. Goltz SR, Campbell WW, Chitchumroonchokchai C, et al. Meal triacylglycerol profile modulates postprandial absorption of carotenoids in humans. *Mol Nutr Food Res.* 2012;56:866–877.

Chapter Five: Nutritarian Boot Camp

1. USDA, Economic Research Service. Food availability (per capita) data system. http://www.ers.usda.gov/data-products/food-availability-(per-capita) -data-system.aspx#.Ud8A6UG1GCk. Lin B-H, Yen ST. The U.S. grain consumption landscape: who eats grain, in what form, where, and how much. USDA Economic Research Service; Economic Research Report No. 50; November 2007; http://www.ers.usda.gov/media/216648/err50_1_.pdf.

2. Halton TL, Willett WC, Liu S, et al. Potato and french fry consumption and risk of type 2 diabetes in women. *Am J Clin Nutr.* 2006;83(2):284–290.

3. Gnagnarella P, Gandini S, La Vecchia C, Maisonneuve P. Glycemic index, glycemic load, and cancer risk: a meta-analysis. *Am J Clin Nutr.* 2008;87(6):1793–1801. Barclay AW, Petocz P, McMillan-Price J, et al. Glycemic index, glycemic load, and chronic disease risk—a meta-analysis of observational studies. *Am J Clin Nutr.* 2008;87(3):627–637.

4. Williams CD, Satia JA, Adair LS, et al. Dietary patterns, food groups, and rectal cancer risk in Whites and African-Americans. *Cancer Epidemiol Biomarkers Prev.* 2009;18(5):1552–1561.

5. Sieri S, Krogh V, Berrino F, et al. Dietary glycemic load and index and risk of coronary heart disease in a large Italian cohort: the EPICOR study. *Arch Intern Med.* 2010;170(7):640–647.

6. Burger KNJ, Beulens JWJ, Boer JMA, et al. Dietary Glycemic Load and Glycemic Index and Risk of Coronary Heart Disease and Stroke in Dutch Men and Women: The EPIC-MORGEN Study. *PLoS One.* 2011;6(10):e25955.

7. Holt S, Brand-Miller J, Petocz P. An insulin index of foods: the insulin demand generated by 1000-Kj portions of common foods. *Am J Clin Nutr.* 1997;66:1264–1276. Bao J, de Jong V, Atkinson F, et al. Food insulin index:

physiologic basis for predicting insulin demand evoked by composite meals. *Am J Clin Nutr.* 2009;90:986–992.

8. Vergnaud AC, Norat T, Romaguera D, et al. Meat consumption and prospective weight change in participants of the EPIC-PANACEA study 1,2,3. *Am J Clin Nutr.* 2010;92(2):398–407. Sabaté J, Ang Y. Nuts and health outcomes: new epidemiologic evidence. *Am J Clin Nutr.* 2009;89(5):1643S–1648S. Fraser GE, Sabaté J, Beeson WL, Strahan TM. A possible protective effect of nut consumption on risk of coronary heart disease: the Adventist Health Study. *Arch Intern Med.* 1992;152(7):1416–1424. Griel AE, Kris-Etherton PM. Tree nuts and the lipid profile: a review of clinical studies. *Br J Nutr.* 2006;96(suppl 2):S68–78. Sabaté J, Oda K, Ros E. Nut consumption and blood lipid levels: a pooled analysis of 25 intervention trials. *Arch Intern Med.* 2010;170(9):821–827. Mattes RD, Kris-Etherton PM, Foster GD. Impact of peanuts and tree nuts on body weight and healthy weight loss in adults. *J Nutr.* 2008;138:1741S–1745S. Bes-Rastrollo M, Sabaté J, Gómez-Gracia E, et al. Nut consumption and weight gain in a Mediterranean cohort: the SUN study. *Obesity.* 2007;15:107–116. Bes-Rastrollo M, Wedick NM, Martínez-González MA, et al. Prospective study of nut consumption, long-term weight change, and obesity risk in women. *Am J Clin Nutr.* 2009;89:1913–1919.

9. Chitnis MM, Yuen JS, Protheroe AS, et al. The type 1 insulin-like growth factor receptor pathway. *Clin Cancer Res.* 2008;14:6364–6370. Werner H, Bruchim I. The insulin-like growth factor-I receptor as an oncogene. *Arch Physiol Biochem.* 2009;115:58–71. Davies M, Gupta S, Goldspink G, et al. The insulin-like growth factor system and colorectal cancer: clinical and experimental evidence. *Int J Colorectal Dis.* 2006;21:201–208. Sandhu MS, Dunger DB, Giovannucci EL. Insulin, insulin-like growth factor-I (IGF-I), IGF binding proteins, their biologic interactions, and colorectal cancer. *J Natl Cancer Inst.* 2002;94:972–980. Rowlands MA, Gunnell D, Harris R, Vatten LJ, Holly JM, Martin RM. Circulating insulin-like growth factor peptides and prostate cancer risk: a systematic review and meta-analysis. *Int J Cancer.* 2009;124(10):2416–2429.

10. Werner H, Bruchim I. The insulin-like growth factor-1 receptor as an oncogene. *Arch Physiol Biochem.* 2009;115(2):58–71. Chitnis MM, Yuen JS, Protheroe AS, et al. The type 1 insulin-like growth factor receptor pathway. *Clin Cancer Res.* 2008;14(20):6364–6370.

11. Bartke A. Minireview: role of the growth hormone/insulin-like growth factor system in mammalian aging. *Endocrinology.* 2005;146:3718–3723.

12. Rinaldi S, Peeters PH, Berrino F, et al. IGF-I, IGFBP-3 and breast cancer risk in women: the European Prospective Investigation into Cancer and Nutrition (EPIC). *Endocr Relat Cancer.* 2006;13:593–605.

13. Hankinson SE, Willett WC, Colditz GA, et al. Circulating concentrations of insulin-like growth factor-I and risk of breast cancer. *Lancet.* 1998;351:1393–1396.

14. Lann D, LeRoith D. The role of endocrine insulin-like growth factor-I and insulin in breast cancer. *J Mammary Gland Biol Neoplasia*. 2008;13:371–379. Allen NE, Roddam AW, Allen DS, et al. A prospective study of serum insulin-like growth factor-I (IGF-I), IGF-II, IGF-binding protein-3 and breast cancer risk. *Br J Cancer*. 2005;92:1283–1287. Fletcher O, Gibson L, Johnson N, et al. Polymorphisms and circulating levels in the insulin-like growth factor system and risk of breast cancer: a systematic review. *Cancer Epidemiol Biomarkers Prev*. 2005;14:2–19. Renehan AG, Zwahlen M, Minder C, et al. Insulin-like growth factor (IGF)-I, IGF binding protein-3, and cancer risk: systematic review and meta-regression analysis *Lancet*. 2004;363(9418):1346–1353. Shi R, Yu H, McLarty J, et al. IGF-I and breast cancer: a meta-analysis. *Int J Cancer*. 2004;111(3):418–423. Sugumar A, Liu YC, Xia Q, et al. Insulin-like growth factor (IGF)-I and IGF-binding protein 3 and the risk of premenopausal breast cancer: a meta-analysis of literature. *Int J Cancer*. 2004;111(2):293–297. Key TJ, Appleby PN, Reeves GK, Roddam AW, Endogenous Hormones and Breast Cancer Collaborative Group. Insulin-like growth factor 1 (IGF1), IGF binding protein 3 (IGFBP3), and breast cancer risk: pooled individual data analysis of 17 prospective studies. *Lancet Oncol*. 2010;11(6):530–542.

15. Vardy ER, Rice PJ, Bowie PC, et al. Increased circulating insulin-like growth factor-1 in late-onset Alzheimer's disease. *J Alzheimers Dis*. 2007;12(4):285–290. Cohen E. Countering neurodegeneration by reducing the activity of the insulin/IGF signaling pathway: current knowledge and future prospects. *Exp Gerontol*. 2011;46(2–3):124–128.

16. Thissen JP, Ketelslegers JM, Underwood LE. Nutritional regulation of the insulin-like growth factors. *Endocr Rev*. 1994;15:80–101. Tsilidis KK, Travis RC, Appleby PN, et al. Insulin-like growth factor pathway genes and blood concentrations, dietary protein and risk of prostate cancer in the NCI Breast and Prostate Cancer Cohort Consortium (BPC3). *Int J Cancer*. 2013;133(2):495–504.

17. Qun LQ, He K, Xu JY. Milk consumption and circulating insulin-like growth factor-1 levels: a systematic literature review. *Int J Food Sci Nutr*. 2009;60(suppl 7):330–340. Heaney RP, McCarron DA, Dawson-Hughes B, et al. Dietary changes favorably affect bone remodeling in older adults. *J Am Diet Assoc*. 1999;99:1228–1233.

18. Roddam AW, Allen NE, Appleby P, et al. Insulin-like growth factors, their binding proteins, and prostate cancer risk: analysis of individual patient data from 12 prospective studies. *Ann Intern Med*. 2008;149(7):461–471. Sim HG, Cheng CW. Changing demography of prostate cancer in Asia. *Eur J Cancer*. 2005;41(6):834–845.

19. Song Y, Chavarro JE, Cao Y, et al. Whole milk intake is associated with prostate cancer-specific mortality among U.S. male physicians *J Nutr*. 2013;143(2):189–196.

20. Giovannucci E, Pollak M, Liu Y, et al. Nutritional predictors of insulin-like growth factor I and their relationships to cancer in men. *Cancer Epidemiol Biomarkers Prev.* 2003;12:84–89. Holmes MD, Pollak MN, Willett WC, et al. Dietary correlates of plasma insulin-like growth factor I and insulin-like growth factor binding protein 3 concentrations. *Cancer Epidemiol Biomarkers Prev.* 2002;11:852–861. Allen NE, Appleby PN, Davey GK, et al. The associations of diet with serum insulin-like growth factor I and its main binding proteins in 292 women meat-eaters, vegetarians, and vegans. *Cancer Epidemiol Biomarkers Prev.* 2002;11:1441–1448. Kaklamani VG, Linos A, Kaklamani E, et al. Dietary fat and carbohydrates are independently associated with circulating insulin-like growth factor 1 and insulin-like growth factor-binding protein 3 concentrations in healthy adults. *J Clin Oncol.* 1999;17:3291–3298. Larsson SC, Wolk K, Brismar K, et al. Association of diet with serum insulin-like growth factor I in middle-aged and elderly men. *Am J Clin Nutr.* 2005;81:1163–1167.

21. Cannata D, Fierz Y, Vijayakumar A, et al. Type 2 diabetes and cancer: what is the connection? *Mt Sinai J Med.* 2010;77:197–213. Venkateswaran V, Haddad AQ, Fleshner NE, et al. Association of diet-induced hyperinsulinemia with accelerated growth of prostate cancer (LNCaP) xenografts. *J Natl Cancer Inst.* 2007;99:1793–1800. Kaaks R. Nutrition, insulin Igf-1 metabolism and cancer risk: a summary of epidemiological evidence. *Novartis Found Symp.* 2004;262:247–260. Discussion 260–268.

22. Dewell A, Weidner G, Sumner MD, et al. Relationship of dietary protein and soy isoflavones to serum Igf-1 and Igf binding protein in the Prostate Cancer Lifestyle Trial. *Nutr Cancer.* 2007;58(1):35–42. Gann PH, Kazer R, Chatterton R, et al. Sequential, randomized trial of a low-fat, high fiber diet and soy supplementation effects on circulating Igf-1 and its binding proteins in premenopausal women. *Int J Cancer.* 2005;116(2):297–303. Khalil DA, Lucas EA, Juma S, et al. Soy protein supplementation increases serum insulin-like growth factor-1 in young and old men but does not affect markers of bone metabolism *J Nutr.* 2002;132(9):2605–2608.

23. Sanderson M, Shu XO, Yu H, et al. Insulin-like growth factor-1, soy protein intake, and breast cancer risk. *Nutr Cancer.* 2004;50(1):8–15. Takata Y, Maskarinec G, Rinaldi S, et al. Serum insulin-like growth factor-1 levels among women in Hawaii and Japan with different levels of tofu intake. *Nutr Cancer.* 2006;56(2):136–142.

24. Salvioli S, Capri M, Bucci L, et al. Why do centenarians escape or postpone cancer? The role of IGF-1, inflammation and p53. *Cancer Immunol Immunother.* 2009;58(12):1909–1917.

25. Crowe FL, Key TJ, Allen NE, et al. The association between diet and serum concentrations of IGF-I, IGFBP-1, IGFBP-2, and IGFBP-3 in the European Prospective Investigation into Cancer and Nutrition. *Cancer Epidemiol.* 2009;18(5):1333–1340. Tsilidis KK, Travis RC, Appleby PN, et al. Insulin-like growth factor pathway genes and blood concentrations, dietary

protein and risk of prostate cancer in the NCI Breast and Prostate Cancer Cohort Consortium (BPC3). *Int J Cancer.* 2013;133(2):495–504.

26. Fontana L, Weiss EP, Holloszy JO. Long-term effects of calorie or protein restriction on serum IGF-1 and IGFBP-3 concentration in humans. *Aging Cell.* 2008;7(5):681–687.

27. Crowe FL, Key TJ, Allen NE, et al. The association between diet and serum concentrations of IGF-I, IGFBP-1, IGFBP-2, and IGFBP-3 in the European Prospective Investigation into Cancer and Nutrition. *Cancer Epidemiol.* 2009;18(5):1333–1340.

28. Fontana L, Klein S, Holloszy JO. Long-term low-protein, low-calorie diet and endurance exercise modulate metabolic factors associated with cancer risk. *Am J Clin Nutr.* 2006;84:1456–1462.

29. Sinha R, Cross AJ, Graubard BI, et al. Meat intake and mortality: a prospective study of over half a million people. *Arch Intern Med.* 2009;169:562–571. Bernstein AM, Sun Q, Hu FB, et al. Major dietary protein sources and risk of coronary heart disease in women. *Circulation.* 2010;122:876–883. Pan A, Sun Q, Bernstein AM, et al. Red meat consumption and mortality: results from 2 prospective cohort studies. *Arch Intern Med.* 2012;172(7):555–663. Ascherio A, Willett WC, Rimm EB, et al. Dietary iron intake and risk of coronary disease among men. *Circulation.* 1994;89:969–974. Larsson SC, Virtamo J, Wolk A. Red meat consumption and risk of stroke in Swedish men. *Am J Clin Nutr.* 2011;94(2):417–421.

30. Tholstrup T, Hjerpsted J, Raff M: Palm olein increases plasma cholesterol moderately compared with olive oil in healthy individuals. *Am J Clin Nutr.* 2011;94:1426–1432. De Oliveira Otto MC, Alonso A, Lee DH, et al. Dietary intakes of zinc and heme iron from red meat, but not from other sources, are associated with greater risk of metabolic syndrome and cardiovascular disease. *J Nutr.* 2012;142:526–533. Ahluwalia N, Genoux A, Ferrieres J, et al. Iron status is associated with carotid atherosclerotic plaques in middle-aged adults. *J Nutr.* 2010;140:812–816. Brewer GJ. Iron and copper toxicity in diseases of aging, particularly atherosclerosis and Alzheimer's disease. *Exp Biol Med.* 2007;232:323–335.

31. Luan DC, Li H, Li SJ, et al. Body iron stores and dietary iron intake in relation to diabetes in adults in North China. *Diabetes Care.* 2008;31:285–286. Rajpathak SN, Crandall JP, Wylie-Rosett J, et al. The role of iron in type 2 diabetes in humans. *Biochim Biophys Acta.* 2009;1790:671–681.

32. Chen GC, Lv DB, Pang Z, et al. Red and processed meat consumption and risk of stroke: a meta-analysis of prospective cohort studies. *Eur J Clin Nutr.* 2013;67:91–95.

33. Kiechl S, Willeit J, Egger G, et al. Body iron stores and the risk of carotid atherosclerosis: prospective results from the Bruneck study. *Circulation.* 1997;96:3300–3307. Steffen LM, Kroenke CH, Yu X, et al. Associations

of plant food, dairy product, and meat intakes with 15-y incidence of elevated blood pressure in young black and white adults: the Coronary Artery Risk Development in Young Adults (CARDIA) Study. *Am J Clin Nutr*. 2005;82:1169–1177; quiz 1363–1364. Tzoulaki I, Brown IJ, Chan Q, et al. Relation of iron and red meat intake to blood pressure: cross sectional epidemiological study. *BMJ*. 2008;337:a258. Wang L, Manson JE, Buring JE, et al. Meat intake and the risk of hypertension in middle-aged and older women. *J Hypertens*. 2008;26:215–222. Miura K, Greenland P, Stamler J, et al. Relation of vegetable, fruit, and meat intake to 7-year blood pressure change in middle-aged men: the Chicago Western Electric Study. *Am J Epidemiol*. 2004;159:572–580.

34. Neish AS. Microbes in gastrointestinal health and disease. *Gastroenterology*. 2009;136:65–80. Backhed F. Host responses to the human microbiome. *Nutr Rev*. 2012;70(suppl 1):S14–17.

35. Koeth RA, Wang Z, Levison BS, et al. Intestinal microbiota metabolism of L-carnitine, a nutrient in red meat, promotes atherosclerosis. *Nat Med*. 2013;19(5):576–585. Wang Z, Klipfell E, Bennett BJ, et al. Gut flora metabolism of phosphatidylcholine promotes cardiovascular disease. *Nature*. 2011;472:57–63. Woolston C. Red meat + wrong bacteria = bad news for hearts. *Nature*. http://www.nature.com/news/red-meat-wrong-bacteria-bad -news-for-hearts-1.12746. Published April 7, 2013. Accessed April 12, 2013.

36. World Cancer Research Fund, American Institute for Cancer Research. Expert report. Food, nutrition, physical activity and the prevention of cancer: a global perspective. World Cancer Research Fund; 2007. Lunn JC, Kuhnle G, Mai V, et al. The effect of haem in red and processed meat on the endogenous formation of N-nitroso compounds in the upper gastrointestinal tract. *Carcinogenesis*. 2007;28:685–690. Kuhnle GG, Story GW, Reda T, et al. Diet-induced endogenous formation of nitroso compounds in the GI tract. *Free Radic Biol Med*. 2007;43:1040–1047. Pan A, Sun Q, Bernstein AM, et al. Red meat consumption and mortality: results from 2 prospective cohort studies. *Arch Intern Med*. 2012;172(7):555–663. Sinha R, Cross AJ, Graubard BI, et al. Meat intake and mortality: a prospective study of over half a million people. *Arch Intern Med*. 2009;169:562–571. Major JM, Cross AJ, Doubeni CA, et al. Socioeconomic deprivation impact on meat intake and mortality: NIH-AARP Diet and Health Study. *Cancer Causes Control*. 2011;22:1699–1707. Key TJ, Fraser GE, Thorogood M, et al. Mortality in vegetarians and nonvegetarians: detailed findings from a collaborative analysis of 5 prospective studies. *Am J Clin Nutr*. 1999;70:516S–524S. Fraser GE. Associations between diet and cancer, ischemic heart disease, and all-cause mortality in non-Hispanic white California Seventh-day Adventists. *Am J Clin Nutr*. 1999;70:532S–538S.

37. Djousse L, Gaziano JM. Egg consumption in relation to cardiovascular disease and mortality: the Physicians' Health Study. *Am J Clin Nutr*. 2008;87:964–969.

38. Djousse L, Gaziano JM, Buring JE, et al. Egg consumption and risk of type 2 diabetes in men and women. *Diabetes Care.* 2009;32:295–300.

39. Trichopoulou A, Psaltopoulou T, Orfanos P, et al. Diet and physical activity in relation to overall mortality amongst adult diabetics in a general population cohort. *J Intern Med.* 2006;259:583–591.

40. Johansson M, Van Guelpen B, Vollset SE, et al. One-carbon metabolism and prostate cancer risk: prospective investigation of seven circulating B vitamins and metabolites. *Cancer Epidemiol Biomarkers Prev.* 2009;18:1538–1543. Platz EA, Clinton SK, Giovannucci E. Association between plasma cholesterol and prostate cancer in the PSA era. *Int J Cancer.* 2008;123:1693–1698.

41. Richman EL, Kenfield SA, Stampfer MJ, et al. Egg, red meat, and poultry intake and risk of lethal prostate cancer in the prostate-specific antigen-era: incidence and survival. *Cancer Prev Res.* 2011;4(12):2110–2121.

42. Richman EL, Kenfield SA, Stampfer MJ, et al. Choline intake and risk of lethal prostate cancer: incidence and survival. *Am J Clin Nutr.* 2012;96:855–863.

43. Zeisel, SH. Choline and brain development. In: Bowman BA, Russell RM, eds. *Present Knowledge in Nutrition.* 9th ed. Washington, DC: International Life Sciences Institute; 2006:352–360. Glunde K, Ackerstaff E, Mori N, et al. Choline phospholipid metabolism in cancer: consequences for molecular pharmaceutical interventions. *Mol Pharm.* 2006;3:496–506. Glunde K, Bhujwalla ZM. Choline kinase alpha in cancer prognosis and treatment. *Lancet Oncol.* 2007;8:855–857.

44. Cho E, Willett WC, Colditz GA, et al. Dietary choline and betaine and the risk of distal colorectal adenoma in women. *J Natl Cancer Inst.* 2007;99:1224–1231.

45. Spence JD, Jenkins DJ, Davignon J. Egg yolk consumption and carotid plaque. *Atherosclerosis.* 2012;224(2):469–473.

46. Hites RA, Foran JA, Carpenter DO, et al. Global assessment of organic contaminants in farmed salmon. *Science.* 2004;303:226–229.

Chapter Six: The Plan

1. Streppel MT, Arends LR, Veer P, et al. Dietary fiber and blood pressure: a meta-analysis of randomized placebo-controlled trials. *Arch Intern Med.* 2005;165:150–156. Lee YP, Puddey IB, Hodgson JM. Protein, Fibre and Blood Pressure: Potential Benefit of Legumes. *Clin Exp Pharmacol Physiol.* 2008;35(4):473–476. Papanikolau Y, Fulgoni VL. Bean Consumption is associated with greater nutrient intake, reduced systolic blood pressure, lower body weight and a smaller waist circumference in adults: Results from the National Health and Nutrition Examination Survey. 1999–2002. *J Am Coll Nutr.* 2008;27(5):569–576.

2. Sievenpiper JL, Kendall CW, Esfahani A, et al. Effect of non-oil-seed pulses on glycaemic control: a systematic review and meta-analysis of randomized controlled experimental trials in people with and without diabetes. *Diabetologia.* 2009;52:1479–1495. Patel A, MacMahon S, Chalmers J, et al. Intensive blood glucose control and vascular outcomes in patients with type 2 diabetes. *N Engl J Med.* 2008;358:2560–2572. Jenkins DA, Kendall CC, Augustin LA, et al. Effect of legumes as part of a low glycemic index diet on glycemic control and cardiovascular risk factors in type 2 diabetes mellitus: a randomized controlled trial. *Arch Intern Med.* 2012;172(21):1653–1660.

3. Bazzano LA, Thompson AM, Tees MT, et al. Non-soy legume consumption lowers cholesterol levels: a meta-analysis of randomized controlled trials. *Nutr Metab Cardiovasc Dis.* 2011;21:94–103.

4. Bednar GE, Patil AR, Murray SM, et al. Starch and fiber fractions in selected food and feed ingredients affect their small intestinal digestibility and fermentability and their large bowel fermentability in vitro in a canine model. *J Nutr.* 2001;131:276–286. Muir JG, O'Dea K. Measurement of resistant starch: factors affecting the amount of starch escaping digestion in vitro. *Am J Clin Nutr.* 1992;56:123–127.

5. Blackberry I, Kouris-Blazos A, Wahlqvist ML, et al. Legumes: the most important dietary predictor of survival in older people of different ethnicities. *Asia Pac J Clin Nutr.* 2004;13(suppl):S126.

6. Weber Lozada K, Keri RA. Bisphenol A increases mammary cancer risk in two distinct mouse models of breast cancer. *Biol Reprod.* 2011;85(3):490–497. Ho S, Tang W, Prins GS, et al. Developmental exposure to estradio and bisphenol-A increases susceptibility to prostate carcinogenesis and epigenetically regulates phosphodiesterase type 4 variant 4. *Cancer Res.* 2006;66:5624–5632. Melzer D, Rice NE, Lewis C, et al. Association of urinary bisphenol A concentration with heart disease: evidence from NHANES 2003/06. *PLoS One.* 2010;5(1):e8673. Lang IA, Galloway TS, Scarlett A, et al. Association of urinary bisphenol A concentration with medical disorders and laboratory abnormalities in adults. *JAMA.* 2008;300(11):1303–1310. Meeker JD, Ehrlich S, Toth TL, et al. Semen quality and sperm DNA damage in relation to urinary bisphenol A among men from an infertility clinic. *Reprod Toxicol.* 2010;30(4):532–539. Brieño-Enríquez MA, Toran N, Martínez F, et al. Gene expression is altered after bisphenol A exposure in human fetal oocytes in vitro. *Mol Hum Reprod.* 2012;18(4):171–183. Sugiura-Ogasawara M, Ozaki Y, Sonta S, Makino T, Suzumori K. Exposure to bisphenol A is associated with recurrent miscarriage. *Human Reprod.* 2005;20:2325–2329. Friedrich MJ. Bisphenol A and reproduction. *JAMA.* 2011;305(1):28. Howdeshell KL, Hotchkiss AK, Thayer KA, et al. Environmental toxins: exposure to bisphenol A advances puberty. *Nature.* 1999;401:763–764. Kiguchi M, Fujita S, Oki H, Shimizu N, Cools AR, Koshikawa N. Behavioural characterisation of rats exposed neonatally to bisphenol-A: responses to a novel environment and to methylphenidate

challenge in a putative model of attention-deficit hyperactivity disorder. *J Neural Trans.* 2008;115(7):1079–1085. Nagel SC, Boechler M, Welshons WV, et al. Relative binding affinity-serum modified access (RBA-SMA) assay predicts the relative in vivo bioactivity of the xenoestrogens bisphenol A and octylphenol. *Environ Health Perspect.* 1997;105(1):70–76. Li D, Zhou Z, Qing Y, et al. Occupational exposure to bisphenol-A (BPA) and the risk of self-reported male sexual dysfunction. *Human Reprod.* 2010;25(2):519–527. Howdeshell KL, Andrew KH, Thayer KA, et al. Environmental toxins: Exposure to bisphenol A advances puberty. *Nature.* 1999;401:763–764. Braun JM, Yolton K, Dietrich KN, et al. Prenatal bisphenol A exposure and early childhood behavior. *Environ Health Perspect.* 2009;117:1945–1952. Carwile JL, Michels KB. Urinary bisphenol A and obesity: NHANES 2003–2006. *Environ Res.* 2011;111(6):825–830. Wang T, Main L, Bing C, et al. Urinary bisphenol a (BPA) concentration associates with obesity and insulin resistance. *J Clin Endocrinol Metab.* 2012;97(2):E223–227. Bhandari R, Xiao J, Shankar A. Urinary bisphenol A and obesity in U.S. children. *Am J Epidemiol.* 2013;177(11):1263–1270.

Appendix: Considering Supplements

1. Pitkin RM. Folate and neural tube defects. *Am J Clin Nutr.* 2007;85:285S–288S.

2. Troen AM, Mitchell B, Sorensen B, et al. Unmetabolized folic acid in plasma is associated with reduced natural killer cell cytotoxicity among postmenopausal women. *J Nutr.* 2006;136:189–194. Smith AD, Kim YI, Refsum H. Is folic acid good for everyone? *Am J Clin Nutr.* 2008;87:517–533. Pfeiffer CM, Caudill SP, Gunter EW, et al. Biochemical indicators of B vitamin status in the US population after folic acid fortification: results from the National Health and Nutrition Examination Survey 1999–2000. *Am J Clin Nutr.* 2005;82:442–450.

3. Charles D, Ness AR, Campbell D, et al. Taking folate in pregnancy and risk of maternal breast cancer. *BMJ.* 2004;329:1375–1376. Figueiredo JC, Grau MV, Haile RW, et al. Folic acid and risk of prostate cancer: results from a randomized clinical trial. *J Natl Cancer Inst.* 2009;101:432–435. Fife J, Raniga S, Hider PN, et al. Folic acid supplementation and colorectal cancer risk: a meta-analysis. *Colorectal Dis.* 2011;13(2):132–137.

4. Stolzenberg-Solomon RZ, Chang SC, Leitzmann MF, et al. Folate intake, alcohol use, and postmenopausal breast cancer risk in the Prostate, Lung, Colorectal, and Ovarian Cancer Screening Trial. *Am J Clin Nutr.* 2006;83:895–904.

5. Baggott JE, Oster RA, Tamura T. Meta-analysis of cancer risk in folic acid supplementation trials. *Cancer Epidemiol.* 2012;36(1):78–81.

6. Figueiredo JC, Grau MV, Haile RW, et al. Folic acid and risk of prostate cancer: results from a randomized clinical trial. *J Natl Cancer Inst.* 2009;101:432–435. Sellers TA, Kushi LH, Cerhan JR, et al. Dietary folate intake, alcohol, and risk of breast cancer in a prospective study of postmenopausal women.

Epidemiology. 2001;12:420–428. Martínez ME, Giovannucci E, Jiang R, et al. Folate fortification, plasma folate, homocysteine and colorectal adenoma recurrence. *Int J Cancer*. 2006;119:1440–1446.

7. Smith AD, Kim YI, Refsum H. Is folic acid good for everyone? *Am J Clin Nutr*. 2008;87:517–533.

8. Whitrow MJ, Moore VM, Rumbold AR, et al. Effect of supplemental folic acid in pregnancy on childhood asthma: a prospective birth cohort study. *Am J Epidemiol*. 2009;170:1486–1493. Haberg SE, London SJ, Stigum H, et al. Folic acid supplements in pregnancy and early childhood respiratory health. *Arch Dis Child*. 2009;94:180–184. Kwan ML, Jensen CD, Block G, et al. Maternal diet and risk of childhood acute lymphoblastic leukemia. *Public Health Rep*. 2009;124:503–514. Petridou E, Ntouvelis E, Dessypris N, et al. Maternal diet and acute lymphoblastic leukemia in young children. *Cancer Epidemiol Biomarkers Prev*. 2005;14:1935–1939. Jensen CD, Block G, Buffler P, et al. Maternal dietary risk factors in childhood acute lymphoblastic leukemia (United States). *Cancer Causes Control*. 2004;15:559–570. Tower RL, Spector LG. The epidemiology of childhood leukemia with a focus on birth weight and diet. *Crit Rev Clin Lab Sci*. 2007;44:203–242. Kallen B. Congenital malformations in infants whose mothers reported the use of folic acid in early pregnancy in Sweden: a prospective population study. *Congenit Anom*. 2007;47:119–124.

9. Higdon J. Carotenoids. In: *An Evidence-Based Approach to Dietary Phytochemicals*. New York: Thieme; 2006: 47–61. Krinsky NI, Johnson EJ. Carotenoid actions and their relation to health and disease. *Mol Aspects Med*. 2005;26:459–516.

10. The Alpha-Tocopherol Beta Carotene Cancer Prevention Study Group. The effect of vitamin E and beta carotene on the incidence of lung cancer and other cancers in male smokers. *N Engl J Med*. 1994;330:1029–1035. Omenn GS, Goodman GE, Thornquist MD, et al. Effects of a combination of beta carotene and vitamin A on lung cancer and cardiovascular disease. *N Engl J Med*. 1996;334:1150–1155.

11. Bjelakovic G, Nikolova D, Gluud LL, et al. Antioxidant supplements for prevention of mortality in healthy participants and patients with various diseases. *Cochrane Database Syst Rev*. 2012;3:CD007176.

12. Mayne ST. Beta-carotene, carotenoids, and disease prevention in humans. *FASEB J*. 1996;10:690–701.

13. Krinsky NI, Johnson EJ. Carotenoid actions and their relation to health and disease. *Mol Aspects Med*. 2005;26:459–516.

14. Melhus H, Michaelsson K, Kindmark A, et al. Excessive dietary intake of vitamin A is associated with reduced bone mineral density and increased risk for hip fracture. *Ann Intern Med*. 1998;129:770–778.

15. Higdon J. Vitamin A. In: *An Evidence-Based Approach to Vitamins and Minerals*. New York: Thieme; 2003; 39–47. Botto LD, Loffredo C, Scanlon KS, et al. Vitamin A and cardiac outflow tract defects. *Epidemiology*. 2001;12:491–496.

16. Bjelakovic G, Nikolova D, Gluud LL, et al. Antioxidant supplements for prevention of mortality in healthy participants and patients with various diseases. *Cochrane Database Syst Rev*. 2012;3:CD007176.

17. Vinceti M, Wei ET, Malagoli C, et al. Adverse health effects of selenium in humans. *Rev Environ Health*. 2001;16:233–251. Mueller AS, Mueller K, Wolf NM, et al. Selenium and diabetes: an enigma? *Free Radic Res*. 2009;43:1029–1059. Navas-Acien A, Bleys J, Guallar E. Selenium intake and cardiovascular risk: what is new? *Curr Opin Lipidol*. 2008;19:43–49. Chan JM, Oh WK, Xie W, et al. Plasma selenium, manganese superoxide dismutase, and intermediate- or high-risk prostate cancer. *J Clin Oncol*. 2009;27:3577–3583.

18. Brewer GJ. Iron and copper toxicity in diseases of aging, particularly atherosclerosis and Alzheimer's disease. *Exp Biol Med*. 2007;232(2):323–335.

19. Morris MC, Evans DA, Tangney CC, et al. Dietary copper and high saturated and trans fat intakes associated with cognitive decline. *Arch Neurol*. 2006;63(8):1085–1088.

20. Office of Dietary Supplements, National Institutes of Health. Dietary supplement fact sheet: vitamin B_{12}. http://ods.od.nih.gov/factsheets/VitaminB_{12}/. Reviewed June 24, 2011.

21. Hooshmand B, Solomon A, Kåreholt I, et al. Homocysteine and holotranscobalamin and the risk of Alzheimer disease: a longitudinal study. *Neurology*. 2010;75:1408–1414. Allen LH. How common is vitamin B_{12} deficiency? *Am J Clin Nutr*. 2009;89:693S–696S.

22. Hyppönen E. Vitamin D and increasing incidence of type 1 diabetes— evidence for an association? *Diabetes Obes Metab*. 2010;12(9):737–743.

23. Holick MF. Sunlight and vitamin D for bone health and prevention of autoimmune diseases, cancers, and cardiovascular disease. *Am J Clin Nutr*. 2004;80:1678S–1688S. Holick MF, Chen TC. Vitamin D deficiency: a worldwide problem with health consequences. *Am J Clin Nutr*. 2008;87:1080S–1086S.

24. Melamed ML, Michos ED, Post W, et al. 25-Hydroxyvitamin D levels and the risk of mortality in the general population. *Arch Intern Med*. 2008;168:1629–1637. Schöttker B, Haug U, Schomburg L, et al. Strong associations of 25-hydroxyvitamin D concentrations with all-cause, cardiovascular, cancer, and respiratory disease mortality in a large cohort study. *Am J Clin Nutr*. 2013;97(4):782–793. Semba RD, Houston DK, Bandinelli S, et al. Relationship of 25-hydroxyvitamin D with all-cause and cardiovascular disease mortality in older community-dwelling adults.

Eur J Clin Nutr. 2010;64:203–209. Zittermann A, Iodice S, Pilz S, et al. Vitamin D deficiency and mortality risk in the general population: a meta-analysis of prospective cohort studies. *Am J Clin Nutr.* 2012;95:91–100.

25. Gandini S, Boniol M, Haukka J, et al. Meta-analysis of observational studies of serum 25-hydroxyvitamin D levels and colorectal, breast and prostate cancer and colorectal adenoma. *Int J Cancer.* 2011;128:1414–1424. Grant WB. Relation between prediagnostic serum 25-hydroxyvitamin D level and incidence of breast, colorectal, and other cancers. *J Photochem Photobiol B.* 2010;101:130–136.

26. Tomson J, Emberson J, Hill M, et al. Vitamin D and risk of death from vascular and non-vascular causes in the Whitehall study and meta-analyses of 12,000 deaths. *Eur Heart J.* 2013;34:1365–1374.

27. Hunt JR. Bioavailability of iron, zinc, and other trace minerals from vegetarian diets. *Am J Clin Nutr.* 2003;78(suppl):633S–639S.

28. De Bortoli MC, Cozzolino SM. Zinc and selenium nutritional status in vegetarians. *Biol Trace Elem Res.* 2009;127(3):228–233. Frassinetti S, Bronzetti G, Caltavuturo L, et al. The role of zinc in life: a review. *J Environ Pathol Toxicol Oncol.* 2006;25(3):597–610. Office of Dietary Supplements, National Institutes of Health. Dietary supplement fact sheet: zinc. http://ods.od.nih.gov/factsheets/Zinc/. Reviewed June 5, 2013.

29. Gonzalez A, Peters U, Lampe JW, White E. Zinc intake from supplements and diet and prostate cancer. *Nutr Cancer.* 2009;61(2):206–215. Whelan P, Walker BE, Kelleher J. Zinc, vitamin A and prostatic cancer. *Br J Urol.* 1983;55:525–528. Ogunlewe JO, Osegbe DN. Zinc and cadmium concentrations in indigenous blacks with normal, hypertrophic, and malignant prostate. *Cancer.* 1989;63:1388–1392. Feustel A, Wennrich R, Schmidt B. Serum-Zn-levels in prostatic cancer. *Urol Res.* 1989;17:41–42.

30. Waldmann A, Koschizke JW, Leitzmann C, Hahn A. Dietary intakes and lifestyle factors of a vegan population in Germany: results from the German Vegan Study. *Eur J Clin Nutr.* 2003;57:947–955. Krajcovicová-Kudláčková M, Bucková K, Klimes I, Seboková E. Iodine deficiency in vegetarians and vegans. *Ann Nutr Metab.* 2003;47(5):183–185.

Acknowledgments

I would like to thank my entire team at DrFuhrman.com, whose work is not merely a job but a passion supporting a mission of caring, enabling so many to improve their health. For this book specifically, Linda Popescu RD, our food scientist, who assists me with nutritional calculations, menu evaluation and scoring, and helped me develop and test the recipes, and Deana Ferreri, Ph.D., our cardiovascular nutritional scientist, who aids me in compiling, evaluating, and comparing research articles and their findings. My wife, Lisa Fuhrman, always helps me with proofreading.

The skilled professional team at HarperOne is always a pleasure to work with. From vice president and executive editor Gideon Weil to production editor Lisa Zuniga and senior director of publicity Melinda Mullin, they are top-notch.

Index

Page numbers in *italics* refer to illustrations.

About the Author

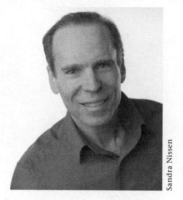

Sandra Nissen

JOEL FUHRMAN, M.D., is a board-certified family physician and nutritional researcher who specializes in preventing and reversing disease through nutritional and natural methods. Dr. Fuhrman is the research director of the Nutritional Research Foundation. He is the author of several books, including the *New York Times* bestsellers *Eat to Live, Eat to Live Cookbook, Super Immunity,* and *The End of Diabetes*. To learn more about the author, visit www.drfuhrman.com.

ALSO BY DR. FUHRMAN

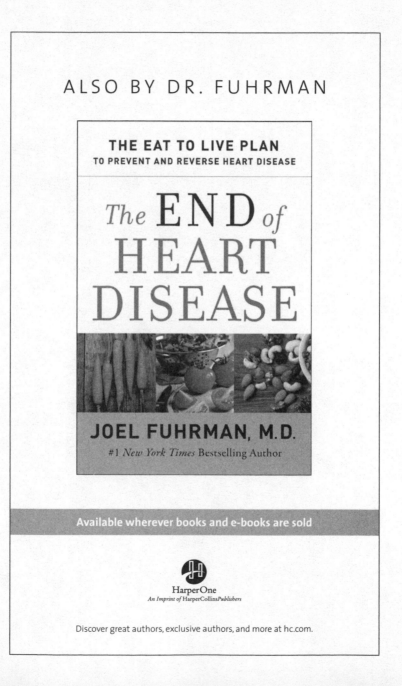

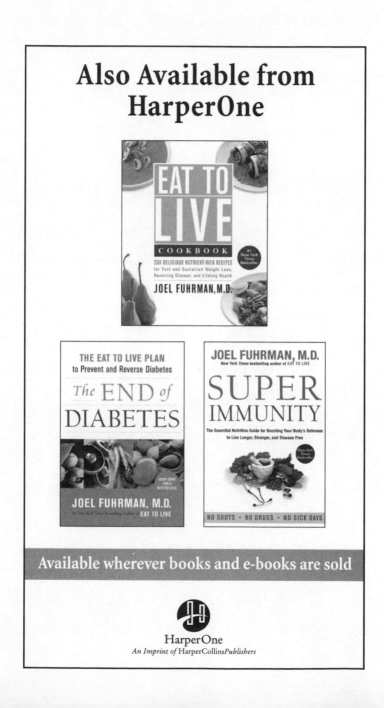